❖

Pregnancy
and
Dreams

❖

Pregnancy and Dreams

How to have a peaceful pregnancy by
understanding your dreams, fantasies,
daydreams and nightmares

❖

Patricia Maybruck, Ph.D.

Foreword by
Patricia Garfield, Ph.D.

JEREMY P. TARCHER, INC.
LOS ANGELES

Library of Congress Cataloging in Publication Data

Maybruck, Patricia.
    Pregnancy and dreams: how to have a peaceful pregnancy by understanding
your dreams, fantasies daydreams, and nightmares/Patricia Maybruck;
foreword by Patricia Garfield.
        p. cm.
    Includes index.
    ISBN 0-87477-512-4.—ISBN 0-87477-522-1 (pbk.)
    1. Pregnancy—Psychological aspects.   2. Dreams.   3. Nightmares.
I. Title.
RG560.M38   1989   89-5124
618.2'4-dc20   CIP

Jeremy P. Tarcher, Inc.
9110 Sunset Blvd.
Los Angeles, CA 90069

Design by Gary Hespenheide

Manufactured in the United States of America
10 9 8 7 6 5 4 3 2 1

First Edition

Dedicated to
the courageous expectant mothers
who made this book possible

CONTENTS

❖

PART ONE
Dreams and Pregnancy

PART TWO
Understanding Your Dreams

PART THREE
Resolving the Six Fears

ACKNOWLEDGMENTS

Whatever I accomplish now and in the future is due to the inspiration of my three mentors, Ross H. Moore, Ph.D.; the late Daniel H. Casriel, M.D.; and Rachel Naomi Remen, M.D. I wish to thank them now for their generosity, wisdom, and love.

My special appreciation to the hundreds of dreaming mothers who were willing to share their innermost thoughts. This book is dedicated to you, because without your help my research would not have been possible. Your courage and determination in the face of often overwhelming anxiety make you shining examples of motherhood. My gratitude also to the expectant fathers. Your input about your mates' and your own dreams was a source of many insights.

Many thanks are due Helen Ballou, Director of Community Education, Napa Valley College, California, for assisting me to reach women in early pregnancy. My appreciation also to all the childbirth preparation instructors who helped me obtain such wonderful volunteers for my research. I particularly remain indebted to Phyllis Dunlavy, Lamaze instructor and obstetrics practitioner at Kaiser-Permanente Hospital, Vallejo, California, for her constant enthusiasm and wise counsel. Thanks are due the many members of the International Childbirth Educators Association who applauded my research findings and who continue to give moral support to the campaign for early prenatal education. My appreciation as well to Bradley childbirth educator and author Carl Jones for his interest and dedication to our common goal of anxiety-free, joyful pregnancies and births.

I am also indebted to the fine journalists Marta Vogel and Mary Roach, whose magazine articles about my work prompted hundreds of expectant women to correspond with me about their dreams and pregnancy experiences. These letters validated my research findings and provided insights into the emotional lives of the contemporary women quoted in this book.

After its initial conception, *Pregnancy and Dreams* would not have happened without the advice and friendship of Theo Gund and Candice Fuhrman, my literary agents, who helped me find the best of all possible publishers, Jeremy P. Tarcher. Jeremy Tarcher was the kind and gentle "physician" in charge, and his executive editor, Hank Stine, the "coach" who guided me through my labors. My gratitude to both of them for making it comparatively painless and for teaching me how to deliver my most pregnant ideas.

I also owe appreciation to the members of the Association for the Study of Dreams for giving me the opportunity to discuss my research with colleagues in the field. My heartfelt thanks to Patricia Garfield, Ph.D., Robert Van de Castle, Ph.D., and Stanley Krippner, Ph.D., who liberally shared their friendship, time, and knowledge of the science of dreams.

Thank you, all my San Francisco and Napa Valley friends of Bill W. Also, members of the San Francisco Professional Women's Network, especially PWN President Angela Coppola. Emotional support from these dear associates nourished me whenever my spirits flagged.

This book could never have been completed without the help and encouragement of my family. Mary C. P.; Heidi and Andrew; Jon and Deki—thanks for your love and the computer assistance; Nyima, Dawa, and Wesley—you are truly "dream babies"; and finally, my dear husband Milton—you continue to make all my dreams come true.

My thanks are due to so many others who helped me give birth to this book that there is no way I can list each one separately. To all who cheered me on in countless ways, my deepest gratitude.

FOREWORD

The grand adventure of pregnancy will be enriched with Patricia Maybruck's remarkable *Pregnancy and Dreams*. Thanks to their hormonal changes, pregnant women dream more often and more vividly than ever. As is true for any traveler in an exotic land, the journey is easier in the company of an experienced guide.

A two-time mother herself, as well as a childbirth educator and a psychologist, Maybruck combines professional skills with the nurturance of a mature and loving woman. In writing *Pregnancy and Dreams,* she drew upon the wisdom of her personal experience of giving birth, the dream diaries of the women in her pregnancy classes, current research, and her own investigation of more than 1,000 dreams from almost seventy pregnant women—the largest and most complete such study to date.

With a sure hand, Maybruck delineates the universal symbols of pregnancy in Part One, revealing their usual meanings and giving the mother-to-be simple techniques for decoding unique or rare dream images. Many readers will find reassurance in the typical pregnancy themes.

Maybruck explains how the majority of the pregnant woman's nightmares relate to one of the six common pregnancy fears: that her child may be unhealthy, that she may be an inadequate parent, that she may lose her mate, that she may have a difficult delivery, that she may lose control, or that she cannot cope financially. Emotional responses to each of these typical fears my be present in the pregnant woman's unpleasant dreams. Maybruck shows how to recognize repressed emotions that appear in dreams, and she sets forth ways to express these feelings, including the surprising means of making sounds.

Maybruck's book covers more than the dreams of pregnancy. It's also about the hopes and fears *behind* those dreams, and about helping the pregnant woman cope with the exaggerated emotions that result from her hormonal upsurges. Beyond that, Maybruck guides the reader in transforming any fearful dreams she might have into joyful, healthful dreaming. By recognizing the common themes and emotions of pregnancy in her own dreams, the woman begins the process of changing negative energy into positive strength. In Part Two, Maybruck gives further methods of converting anxiety and other negative emotions into supportive affirmations, positive daydreams, and preplanned night dreams—all of which nourish the woman's inner child and, hence, her unborn child.

The entire book, especially Part Three, is packed with practical suggestions for enhancing the pregnant woman's ability to relax, to set her mind at ease about the six major causes of worry during childbearing, and to release and ride her "birthing energy." She offers special ways for the pregnant woman and her mate to intimately share the experience of childbirth.

As a clinical psychologist and the author of *Creative Dreaming,* I have long advocated the value of the dreamer taking action in frightening dreams. Maybruck relates how those pregnant women in her study who managed to behave assertively in their dreams of danger had shorter labors (less than ten hours) than those who did not behave assertively. This is good news for pregnant women, especially when the means to accomplish these changes in dreams is given so clearly and succinctly.

A mother myself—and now a grandmother—I know, too, how useful this guidebook will be to generations of women to come. Maybruck provides almost everything the pregnant woman needs to know about her emotions prior to entering childbirth preparation class, and enhances the information of those who are already enrolled. Some of her advice will be treasured during the postpartum period, and possibly for years afterward—particularly the sections on recognizing and expressing emotions and using creative daydreaming to improve the quality of waking life.

When a woman is pregnant her dream life expands, as I've described in my recent *Women's Bodies, Women's Dreams*. Each of her dreams, even the alarming ones, are friends to be welcomed. They teach her about her hidden emotions and give her the opportunity to renew her life. With Patricia Maybruck's dream guidebook in hand, many pregnant women will have a happier and healthier pregnancy.

Patricia Garfield, Ph.D.
San Francisco, August 1989

INTRODUCTION

This book is the fulfillment of a dream of my own, to help contemporary couples alleviate the needless anxiety and pain they undergo during pregnancy.

At the age of fifty-six, after working as a family therapist for many years, I entered San Francisco's Saybrook Institute for graduate work in the psychology of pregnancy and childbirth. When the expectant women I was studying resisted sharing their feelings with me, I hit upon the idea of studying their dreams.

Most people think of a dream as something "outside" themselves that "happens" to them in their sleep. The retelling of a dream is similar to describing a movie we saw recently, or a book we just read. When reporting such a vision, we tend to forget that we ourselves created it, and that its components are probably drawn from our own perceptions, memories, and experiences. By gently encouraging expectant parents to discuss their dreams, I found it remarkably easy to persuade them to confide their formerly secret attitudes and emotions.

When I began my doctoral studies, one of the professors on my dissertation committee was Stanley Krippner, Ph.D., who had conducted a small study of pregnant women's dreams in 1974. With encouragement from Dr. Krippner and two other professors on my committee, I started my own investigation of expectant mothers' dreams and attitudes. The resulting doctoral study took more than two years and included in-depth personal interviews and a comprehensive analysis of more than 1,000 dream records from seventy women in various stages of pregnancy.

These participants were much more anxious than anyone might have suspected. Preliminary questionnaires filled out by each subject addressed the topics of health, childbirth, and parenting. Only two of the seventy women said they had any negative feelings about being pregnant, and just twenty-eight admitted to outright fears about pregnancy and childbirth. Yet, 419 (forty percent) of the total dreams collected from all subjects were nightmares reflecting emotions that ranged from fear to abject terror.

Most of the participants came from the dozens of childbirth preparation classes I visited in California's Napa Valley. Others answered newspaper ads or heard about the project and volunteered. Three women dropped out of the study, saying that the recording process proved too stressful; instead, they preferred to forget their nightmares. These three cases enabled me to reassure the other participants that writing their dream reports actually could *ease* the anxiety such memories might evoke. Furthermore, all volunteers were encouraged to call me for free counseling should the need arise.

The remaining sixty-seven participants claimed varying ages and backgrounds. Forty-nine of the women were in their first pregnancies (primiparae); eighteen had one or more children (multiparae). Every participant signed a release guaranteeing them anonymity when I published my findings.

It became quite evident early in the project that I had set a difficult task for myself. As long ago as 1945, Dr. Helene Deutsch, a pioneer in female psychology and author of *The Psychology of Women,* had written that expectant mothers appear to turn inward, and even those who usually are quite outgoing seem to regress to a childlike demureness when pregnant. In 1971 the psychologist Dr. Robert Van de Castle speculated that this reluctance to talk about feelings—or dreams—might be due to the woman's fear of ridicule or being judged an inadequate mother.

Besides these long-known traits of pregnancy, I had to deal with my volunteers' lack of motivation or desire to commit themselves to new projects. To encourage them to continue the study, I presented a small layette gift to anyone who submitted twelve dream reports. I also made contact with all participants through weekly phone calls and postcards. This personal touch helped develop a climate of trust and enthusiasm possibly missing in previous studies of pregnant women.

The principal reason earlier works have not received more serious attention is that they assessed such small samples. For instance, in 1968 Van de Castle and Peggy Kinder analyzed dreams from only fourteen pregnant women; four years later, Dr. Stanley Krippner and others examined eleven subjects; and Dr. Judith Ballou evaluated twelve and Dr. Cecelia Jones, thirteen, in 1978. In 1985, journalist Eileen Stukane summarized most previous research in *The Dream Worlds of Pregnancy*. Stukane quoted Van de Castle at length, as well as the comments of pregnant women she interviewed personally. My doctoral study explored more than 1,000 dreams from sixty-seven pregnant women and is so much larger than the earlier psychologists' investigations, that its findings appear to be more definitive.

My investigation also revealed that expectant mothers who were able to be assertive in their frightening dreams— to defend themselves or call for help—had significantly shorter labors than did those who were consistently victimized in their nightmares. This discovery led to my development of new techniques that have been of great benefit to many pregnant women.

Yet, when I first reported my findings, there were some negative reactions. One childbirth educator accused me of being an alarmist about an ideally carefree and optimistic period in women's lives. My reply was that I strictly adhered to the facts. Rather than ignoring evidence of high anxiety among expectant parents, it is only common sense—and sound psychological therapy—to encourage them to communicate their fears. An open approach reduces the tension that has potentially harmful repercussions.

When people are undergoing other transitions—the death of a loved one, divorce, or even stress on the job—physicians and psychologists willingly offer helpful remedies and advice. Yet, many in the obstetrical field continue to belittle the pregnant woman's inner struggles; their typical response has been that a certain amount of anxiety is necessary in order for a woman to take seriously her impending role as a mother. In 1982, the well-known pediatrician T. Berry Brazelton made such an argument in *Parent-Infant Bonding*, by Dr. Marshall Klaus and Dr. John H. Kennell, a book which in other respects decries the increasing tendency of the medical community to intervene in the natural process of pregnancy and childbirth.

Absence of anxiety and stress is essential in childbirth. Obstetricians have known this for decades. Dr. Grantley Dick-Read first advocated natural delivery methods in 1933 with his then-controversial *Childbirth Without Fear*. The book emphasized relaxation as an antidote to labor pains. In 1962 Dr. J. V. Kelly presented the *American Journal of Obstetrics and Gynecology* with evidence which suggested that when women are afraid or anxious, tension causes the uterus to contract more slowly, resulting in longer labor. If a woman has been nervous during most of her pregnancy, it's unrealistic to expect her to suddenly become relaxed when labor begins.

Expectant parents deserve to know all the common techniques for stress avoidance available during possible crisis situations. They have a right to probe every advantage and disadvantage of the new technology and to make educated choices about their interventions in what remains an essentially normal, healthy process. Pregnancy and childbirth ought to be times of joy and fulfillment, when both parents are lovingly bonded by the miracle of the life they bring forth. Instead, this transition all too often evokes confusion, pain, and needless anxiety.

Even more important, in my opinion, there is growing evidence that anxiety, tension, and stress in the pregnant woman *also are experienced by the unborn child.* Medical research by Drs. Antonio J. Ferreira, Albert Liley, and many others indicates that the biochemical changes taking place within the mother extend to the fetus via the placenta. When the pregnant woman is anxious, measurable increases in adrenalin, stomach secretions, and additional body changes cause definitive negative reactions in the unborn child.

The harmful effects on the fetus of ingested chemicals (nicotine, alcohol, recreational substances, certain prescription drugs, and anesthetics) have been widely publicized. Yet, health professionals say comparatively little about the dangerous chemicals the expectant mother's own body produces when she is anxious or stressed.

Until recently, most practitioners have also failed to explore the relationship between a woman's feelings during pregnancy and her infant's future personality. In *The Secret Life of the Unborn Child,* Dr. Thomas Verny provides evidence that the fetus, at least by the sixth month, has the same reflexes and responses to touch, sound, and light as the newborn. Therefore, the baby is not a "blank slate" awaiting the programming of caregivers and environment. On the contrary, Dr. Marshall Klaus in *The Amazing Newborn* tells us that immediately after birth the infant is capable of recognizing its parents' voices and touch. The baby also exhibits decided preferences for a variety of stimuli, from types of music to specific positions in which it likes to be held.

My experience with clients who have regressed under hypnosis to early infancy and even *in utero* memories has convinced me that the unborn child does know when it is loved, wanted, and accepted. While this places a heavier responsibility on the parents, it also provides a wonderful opportunity for them to help their baby come into this world feeling welcomed and nurtured.

After completing my doctoral investigation, I began publicizing my findings and teaching classes for couples in early pregnancy. Articles in *Parents, Working Mother, Self,* and *Hippocrates* magazines yielded thousands of letters from expectant mothers and fathers about unusual dreams and other extraordinary consciousness experiences. This correspondence greatly substantiated my preliminary conclusions, since each writer spoke of nightmares similar to those experienced by my subjects. In addition, those writers expressed relief upon discovering the commonality of their dreams and reactions.

Finally, women came forward at lectures, workshops, and classes to tell me that their own experiences paralleled those described in my doctoral investigation. All were eager to know how they could use their dreams to relieve stress. Many confided that they feared they were abnormal and had not even admitted these doubts to themselves. When I lectured at a 1987 convention of the International Childbirth Educators Association in Los Angeles, a number of participants applauded my efforts to convince obstetrical professionals that pregnant women are experiencing high levels of unexpressed anxiety, a condition demanding serious attention.

Many possible explanations exist for the repressed tension found in my subjects. The primary reasons are a stressful environment, belief in "old wives' tales," and the so-called Superwoman Syndrome.

Could it be that the women whose dreams I collected happened to be exposed to unusual circumstances or an especially stressful environment? No, this definitely was not the case. The majority of my volunteers lived in the suburban and rural areas of California's serene Napa Valley, a region boasting some of the nation's most advanced obstetrical facilities. Even low-income couples residing there can attend free childbirth preparation classes and receive the same hospital care as their more affluent neighbors.

Perhaps contemporary women have been "brainwashed" by some of the old myths surrounding pregnancy as well as by the emergence of the Superwoman Syndrome. Admissions of fear or doubt about pregnancy, they believe, somehow will lead to disgrace in the eyes of their peers, mates, and obstetrical personnel. Modern women also are constantly reminded that they have many advantages denied their mothers and grandmothers; they consequently ignore or repress worries and fears.

Some expectant mothers may have been indoctrinated with the old wives' tale about negative thoughts and their adverse effect on pregnancy. Reality differs: it is the *repression* of fears or negativity that leads to tension and stress. If not confronted, these conditions may eventually cause increased levels of anxiety and illness.

As my investigation got under way, I discovered other reasons for unusually high anxiety among pregnant women:

- Normal physiological changes
- Normal mood swings
- Lack of emotional support
- Misinformation about new obstetrical technology
- Pregnancy after age thirty
- Balancing career and motherhood

Pregnancy is a time of drastic bodily changes that normally cause a certain amount of upset. Rapid shifts in hormonal balance account for stomach distress, frequent urination, sleep disturbances, and, occasionally, emotional confusion. Many women experience extreme mood swings during early pregnancy so that they may feel weepy or irritable one moment and blissfully happy the next. As the body adjusts by the second trimester, most of these conditions fade or disappear completely. None of this is news; expectant mothers have complained of these symptoms for generations.

Although pregnant women have always experienced a

certain amount of anxiety, their fears loom larger today because of misinformation about the dangers and side effects of new medical technology such as fetal monitoring, sonograms, and amniocentesis. Furthermore, childbearing women are older now than ever before. This probably results from their increased presence in the labor force and the postponement of pregnancy until careers are launched and finances more secure. When these women do conceive, they often learn that birth defects and complications are more likely after age thirty. Therefore, it becomes obvious that pregnancy in today's world has all the ingredients for an anxiety-provoking experience. Those who complain are often told to be patient, that these worries are temporary, and that all will be forgotten once the baby is born. I believe this patronizing attitude unfairly minimizes the pregnant woman's need to be taken seriously.

Today's expectant mother needs more than medical and economic assistance. She also requires emotional support and peace of mind. If she's married, the pregnant woman usually turns to her husband for comfort, but all too often he himself is beset with stress and uncertainty. Traditionally, she also has sought reassurances from her mother, other female relatives, and friends. Yet, the pregnant woman's relationship with her mother sometimes remains scarred from the wounds of adolescent conflicts. The normal process of growing up happens very rapidly in today's society; young women hurry off to college or jobs, then to marriage or live-in relationships, often carrying with them uncompleted issues which might have been resolved had they stayed at home or received counseling about these conflicts. The result is that many childbearing women still harbor resentments and feel uneasy about confiding in their mothers or opening themselves to possible parental disapproval or control.

Moreover, today's expectant mother often lacks female relatives or friends who might lend support. Other women appear less available in our nuclear society, and many refuse to discuss their worries, fearing ridicule or some other harsh judgment.

The expectant mother formerly turned to her obstetrician for information and reassurances, but modern doctors are frequently too busy or not interested in emotional matters. Furthermore, many pregnant women now use group medical plans that provide basic care at the cost of personal attention. Patients frequently consult different doctors at each monthly check-up and sometimes remain ignorant (until going into labor) of which one will be delivering the baby.

Of course, prenatal childbirth workshops exist. But while the instructor may spend considerable time putting to rest fears and anxieties, most women are not admitted to such classes until the third trimester and many are so close to delivery that they're unable to complete the series. Thus, American women undergo six months or more of emotional upheaval before receiving even this minimal amount of psychological support.

As I began to help expectant couples deal with the stress preventing them from enjoying the unique pleasures of pregnancy, a system for resolving the underlying anxieties gradually evolved. The result—a simple, five-step program for understanding dreams and other states of consciousness—is presented in this book. The five steps include

- Keeping a dream diary
- Understanding dream symbols and diagramming your dreams
- Understanding your emotions
- Interpreting your dreams
- Controlling your dreams

Once you have mastered this easy program, you will be prepared to learn about the other fascinating states of consciousness many pregnant women experience, including daydreams and fantasies, hypnagogic and trance states, visions, and out-of-body sensations.

Extreme hormonal shifts may explain some of these occurrences in expectant mothers. Many of my students feared they were going insane or worried that there might be something terribly wrong with their unborn babies until they discovered that these phenomena are more likely to happen during pregnancy than at any other time. Whatever the cause, unusual states do not indicate insanity or abnormality. Moreover, they can be controlled and employed to enhance feelings of well-being and health. This book will teach you how to use these powerful mental abilities to make the transition from pregnancy to childbirth fulfilling and joyful.

If you are one of the courageous women who has decided to become a single parent, this book is also for you. When you learn to understand your dreams—even the scary ones—you can get in touch with yourself, ease anxiety, and gain the self-confidence necessary to help you embark on this glorious adventure. As a single woman, you already may have found a friend willing to act as your "coach" and partner during labor. Don't be surprised if he or she also has unusual dreams, directly related to your pregnancy and the coming event.

Finally, this book will be of great value for the father-to-be. My work with expectant parents indicated that many men experience dreams and nightmares remarkably similar to those of their pregnant wives. Although their dreams are less intense, future dads nevertheless endure unexpressed anxiety about their impending roles. Each chapter in this book includes information on how emotional states change during the course of pregnancy, with tips on the ways both of you can use your dreams, visions, and fantasies to deepen your love for each other and prepare for the new family.

One fascinating trait of expectant dads' dreams is that they sometimes seem to be telepathic. I discovered this phenomenon accidentally when the husband of one of my volunteers told me, "Last night I had a dream that was almost exactly like my wife's." Some of the couples in my prenatal classes have learned to use these dreams, which I have dubbed "symbiotic," to gain insights into their relationships and to give each other emotional support during times of stress.

The dreams, daydreams, and other unusual consciousness experiences quoted in this book are taken from actual diaries, dream journals, and tape-recorded interviews with hundreds of expectant parents. Subjects include the volunteers from my doctoral investigation; correspondents who read about my work in national magazines; students in my Early Pregnancy, Dreams During Pregnancy, and Relaxation in Pregnancy classes; and counseling clients. To protect confidentiality, I have changed the names and, in a few cases, some identifying descriptions. Otherwise, the quotes are accurate. Since my subjects come from such varying backgrounds, I believe their experiences can be generalized to most American expectant parents.

It's best to read this book one chapter at a time, following the suggestions in each chapter before proceeding to the next. Absorbing this book in solitude, pregnant women can achieve amazing results by using my five-step program for understanding their dreams and fantasies—but it's more fun and much more effective if couples study together. Expectant parents in my California-based prenatal classes report that taking a few minutes each day to share dream experiences has strengthened their relationship.

Having a baby can and ought to be a fun-filled, exciting adventure, but frightening dreams and anxieties often make it a living nightmare. My purpose, my mission, is to assist in breaking this pattern. I seek to remove fear and pain from the experience of pregnancy and childbirth, replacing negativity with the powerful forces of love and acceptance. Only in this way can parents help their infants begin life with trust and the total, unconditional love and nurturance they need to develop into confident, self-actualized adults.

It is my hope that this book, which contains the information and techniques that have helped so many pregnant women achieve joyful and fulfilling pregnancies, will provide relief for the thousands of couples who are still suffering needless anxiety about life's most miraculous adventure.

PART ONE

❖

Dreams

❖

and

❖

Pregnancy

❖

CHAPTER 1

❖

Dreams and the Pregnant Mind

In the fourth month of her first pregnancy, Robyn had this dream:

> I am swimming in the ocean, trying to get to the shore. There's a strong undertow that keeps me from going very far but I'm not worried. The water feels pleasantly warm and I'm only a few yards from a house which is built right out into the water. Somehow I know I'll get to the house eventually. It's a big, two-story, shingled house, and I can see every detail—even the nail heads in the shingles. Then I notice my mother looking out one of the windows. She's smiling and waving to me. Next I notice the water around me is *full* of turtles of all kinds! Most are huge and they're swimming right along beside me. Then I woke up, feeling quite puzzled about this weird dream!

If you are expecting a baby, you probably have been dreaming more than usual. Like Robyn, you may be noticing vivid details and puzzling or bizarre episodes. Your dreams often appear to contain disturbing or nightmarish qualities. All these nightly adventures are a perfectly normal characteristic of pregnancy.

The Unique Qualities of Pregnant Women's Dreams

Krippner, Van de Castle, and many other researchers who study sleep patterns have known for decades that expectant mothers' dreams are remarkably different from those of nonpregnant women. Not only do expectant mothers dream more vividly, but they also are able to recall these dreams more easily than was the case before they conceived.

Although dream research has made great strides since the 1950s, much continues to remain a mystery. Since 1965 when Dr. David Cheek, a well-known obstetrician and hypnotherapist, reported on his patients' dreams, at least a dozen other scientists have attempted to define this subject. My 1986 study was the largest and probably most in-depth investigation of pregnancy and dreams.

Still, we do not know exactly why expectant women dream so vividly or why they are able to remember their dreams more easily than any other group. Contemporary scientists can only theorize about the reasons for the intensity and extraordinary content of these dreams.

WHY DREAMS DURING PREGNANCY ARE DIFFERENT

Several theories attempt to explain the unusual traits of pregnancy dreams. One holds that the extreme hormonal changes occurring in pregnancy correlate with certain biochemical levels present during the dreaming state. Another theory links the irregular sleep patterns of most expectant mothers with better dream recall, simply because the women awaken more frequently. A third theory emphasizes the fact that everyone—female or male, pregnant or nonpregnant—has remarkably different dreams while going through any type of transition or life crisis, such as marriage, divorce, changing jobs, moving, or pregnancy and childbirth. Finally, all three of these concepts may be working together at various times during the pregnancy.

The first theory, that hormonal changes affect pregnancy dreams, has not yet been substantiated. Neurophysiologists, scientists who examine the physical aspects of the mind and brain, continue to investigate the nature of the biochemical changes occurring during dreaming. In the future these researchers may be able to offer data that the increased levels of certain hormones found during pregnancy are also present in smaller amounts when nonpregnant people dream.

The second theory does not provide much new information. It is true that expectant mothers' sleep patterns are quite different than those of most other women. As long ago as 1969, Dr. I. Karacan and a group of other prominent researchers and dream psychologists conducted two carefully monitored investigations, indicating that an uninterrupted night's rest during pregnancy is rare. (This is especially so during the last trimester, when the pressure of the enlarged uterus on the bladder necessitates frequent trips to the bathroom.) It seems logical that numerous awakenings would help anyone recall dreams more easily. Yet, this theory does not explain the unusual content of pregnancy dreams. For example, a seasoned dream psychologist can identify certain dreams as being the creations of a pregnant mind—sometimes when the patient's physician does not know that she is expecting.

The third supposition, suggesting that any transition of life-crisis proportions will be reflected in dreams, appears to come closest to explaining the unusual nature of pregnant women's dreams. One long-standing, reliable theory about dreams in general is that they tend to mirror the subject's personality and concerns while awake. This third explanation also accounts for the distinctly different dreams pregnant women experience during each trimester. Since each three-month interval is accompanied by different physical changes, both in the fetus and in the mother's body, dream patterns would change accordingly.

THE SPECIAL DREAM SYMBOLS OF PREGNANCY

Carrying this reasoning a step farther, the transition theory might explain the remarkable fact that pregnant women's dreams contain the same or similar symbols and elements. For instance, nearly all of these dreams make some reference to water, thought to be a symbol of pregnancy and birth.

Robyn's dream, quoted at the beginning of this chapter, took place in an ocean setting typical of second and third trimester dreams. Interestingly, this dream gives almost no clues as to other facts about Robyn. She is a secretary who works part-time as an aerobics instructor, yet her dream indicates the most pressing aspect of her life: impending motherhood.

A significant number of pregnancy dreams depict amphibians, such as lizards or the turtles described by Robyn. Others portray little animals—furry, cuddly bunnies, kittens, or puppies. These small life forms appear to represent the fetus.

Pregnant women frequently dream about their mothers, possibly as a symbol of themselves or maybe as a reminder of unresolved familial conflicts that need to be addressed before enjoying a new role. While Robyn's dream portrays her mother looking out the window, it doesn't seem to indicate any discord. Rather, the parental figure is smiling and waving in a supportive, encouraging manner.

Most dreams during pregnancy depict some type of architecture, believed to represent the expectant woman's body or uterus, the space within. Had I not known Robyn personally, I might have guessed from her dream that she was in her second trimester. She mentions swimming toward a big house with two stories. If Robyn were still in the first three months of her pregnancy, it is likely that the setting would have been smaller and more confined. Note that the mention of a two-story house also might indicate the second trimester.

Dream symbols may change in size and appearance as the

pregnancy progresses, probably because they represent either the growing fetus or the expanding body. Yet the same symbols reappear in each trimester as important clues to the dream's meaning.

For example, the small kittens present during the first three months may turn into panthers or lions in later stages of pregnancy. The initially tiny lizards and mice of Robyn's first trimester eventually become huge turtles. Small rooms similarly give way to larger buildings (such as Robyn's big, two-story house) and even skyscrapers toward the end of pregnancy. Although the details and size may be different, the symbols serve as references to the dreamer's perception of her body.

POSITIVE AND NEGATIVE DREAMS

Some dreams are quite positive and are a natural outgrowth of the desire to see future life and display feelings of love and warmth toward the developing child. More negative dreams may reflect normal concerns about the baby's health and the changes pregnancy is bound to cause in one's life.

An example of the first style, the positive dream, was given to me by Carolyn, general manager of the offices of a large Northern California trucking company. She had the following dream during her second month of pregnancy:

> Dreamt I heard a scratching noise on my bedroom door, so I got up to see what it was. (This was so real, it seemed I had actually [awakened] and heard the sound!) There on the floor by the door was a basket with a tiny baby kitten in it. The poor little thing was all wet and cold, mewing and crying so it sounded more like a baby than a cat. I picked it up and it was shivering so I took it back to bed with me. It snuggled up between my breasts and started sucking on my nipple. This seemed okay in the dream. As it got warm and dry, I fluffed up its fur and it began to purr. It was so cute! I just adored this darling little bit of fluff. Then we both fell asleep. When I really woke up, I

had a hard time believing this was a dream. I know it sounds silly now, but I actually searched under the covers to see if there was a real kitten there!

When Carolyn told her story in one of my Early Pregnancy classes, she discovered that most of the other students had experienced similar dreams. Learning that dreams of small animals are common during pregnancy and that they indicate a desire to comfort and nourish the unborn child, Carolyn appeared quite relieved. "I thought maybe there was something abnormal about me," she admitted. "But while I was actually having the dream, it was wonderful. It was just that part about nursing the kitten that bothered me later."

While many have sweet dreams such as Carolyn's, expectant mothers' dreams consistently show more anxiety and fear than those of other women. In fact, the disturbing dreams greatly outweigh the happy, positive ones. Forty percent of all the dreams analyzed in my study were nightmares from which the women awoke feeling terrified and upset. Another thirty percent contained anxiety-producing elements: hostile or threatening characters, environmental disasters (storms, fires, or earthquakes), and catastrophes such as deaths or funerals. In other words, seventy percent of the 1,048 dreams proved to be negative and indicated anxiety.

This is a startling statistic. Dr. Ernest Hartmann, professor of psychiatry at Tufts University School of Medicine and author of *The Nightmare,* says that no more than one in every 200 adults has nightmares on a regular basis. In order to study the sufferers, Hartman had to select people he characterized as an extreme group, atypical of the general population. However, his investigations did not include pregnant women.

In 1978, psychologists, Dr. Cecilia Jones and Dr. Judith Ballou, focused on expectant mothers in two separate studies. Both noted the similarity of their subjects' dreams as to symbols and theme, yet neither study indicated an unusually high percentage of nightmares. However, in 1980, after closely following nineteen women throughout their first pregnancies, Dr. Myra Leifer concluded that childbirth in the United States had become an experience of anxiety and pain. She also noted that the dreams of her subjects went through identifiable stages as their pregnancies progressed, and that many of these dreams were frightening in quality.

Psychologists and sleep researchers already have established the connection between dreams and life's concerns. If pregnant women's nightmares reflect their true waking states, it seems logical to conclude that many pregnant women are currently experiencing much more anxiety than mothers-to-be did a generation ago.

Anxiety, Stress, and Health during Pregnancy

Does having more nightmares mean that you are on the verge of a nervous breakdown or that you need psychiatric care? Most likely, the answer is no. However, you could suffer from tension that might affect both your and your baby's health.

There is no possible way to avoid stress entirely. Psychologist Suzanne Kobasa of the University of Chicago points out that the only way to maintain an anxiety-free state is to never change jobs, move, marry, or have a child. Probably the only people completely free of stress are either dead or comatose! On the other hand, many people go through all these transitions without ill effects. The important factor is not the avoidance of stress. It is how we deal with it.

In recent years the harmful effects of stress have received much attention from the media, physicians, and psychologists. Yet this connection between mind and body has not been given equal time vis-à-vis pregnancy. If you're expecting a baby, it is of vital importance for you to learn to recognize and cope with the symptoms of stress. Its ill effects on pregnant women's health are

- High blood pressure, nausea, headaches
- Sleep disturbances, insomnia
- Fatigue, irritability, depression
- Miscarriage

High blood pressure is an early symptom of the most commonly dreaded complication of pregnancy, toxemia. Although elevated blood pressure (hypertension) can be due to many other, less alarming problems, it serves notice that something is not normal. Dr. Thomas Brewer, in *What Every Pregnant Woman Should Know*, emphasizes proper diet as the key to prevention of toxemia. Studies are now being done to determine the relationship between anxiety and toxemia. Since high blood pressure itself can lead to a variety of complications, it makes sense for every pregnant woman to know how to identify and relieve tension in her body.

Nausea and headaches, like hypertension, are symptoms of toxemia and many other diseases. They also appear to be such a common complaint during pregnancy that some obstetricians shrug them off. Yet, persistent "morning sickness" could indicate improper nutrition. Stress and anxiety definitely worsen nausea and headaches, and sometimes may be the only direct cause. Dr. Brewer advises eating small amounts of protein during the night to keep the blood sugar level high. I add that the sooner you learn to dispel your subconscious fears, the less likely you are to have nausea or headaches. However, if severe morning sickness continues at other times, to the extent that you're unable to get proper nourishment for yourself and the fetus, insist upon your physician's counsel and serious attention.

Another stress-related symptom to manifest itself during pregnancy is muscle tension. For example, repression of anger causes abdominal muscles to tighten, sometimes leading to heartburn, indigestion, or stomach cramps. Holding back tears restricts throat muscles and forces the toxins normally expelled in the tears to drain into sinuses, ear canals, and the throat. Various infections subsequently result. Muscle tension also prevents the flow of oxygen to that part of the body, rendering a tired and depressed feeling. Additionally, a very complex array of other physical reactions take place, including an increased flow of stomach acid and adrenalin. All of these body alterations cause marked changes in mood and emotions.

A number of medical researchers have investigated the relationship between anxiety and high-risk pregnancies. Women with a history of spontaneous abortions (miscarriages) or special handicaps are often termed high-risk patients. Obstetrician David Cheek tried hypnotizing such patients, suggesting that they telephone him when they were anxious or overwrought by frightening dreams or nightmares. Cheek reported that a significant percentage of these patients had uncomplicated pregnancies and delivered normally. This report of solicitous care was published nearly two decades ago. Unfortunately, many of today's obstetricians lack the time and training to deal with today's accelerated levels of anxiety.

THE ANXIETY TRAP OF MODERN PREGNANCY

There are a number of reasons why contemporary parents-to-be are more tension-prone than were Cheek's high-risk patients or the healthy, low-risk women studied by Ballou and Jones in 1978. They include

- Superwoman Syndrome
- Less emotional support
- Conflicts over careers and motherhood
- Inflated national economy
- New prenatal technology; medical intervention

The Superwoman Syndrome emerged during the 1980s when many women were trying to be all things—successful careerists, expert homemakers, mothers, wives, lovers, and gracious hostesses to their mates' and their own business associates. The result was a strain on their health and emotional well-being. Add to these pressures the sudden hormonal changes of pregnancy and one can identify the anxiety and pain Leifer noticed in her 1980 study.

Women who try to present a Superwoman image to the world are reluctant to admit, even to their mates and friends, that they experience the normal emotional upheaval of pregnancy. Even mothers-to-be who do not work outside the home often believe they should maintain a serene exterior. This repression increases the stress they're already feeling.

Certainly the women's movement of the 1970s has helped many women attain new career heights formerly open only to men. Yet this new freedom is often a trap, bringing with it a host of problems. While there are more women in the work force than ever before, a large number have had to make hard choices between careers and families. Others have postponed childbearing until their "biological clocks" almost run out; fears of defective babies and difficult, complicated delivery then surface. Others not wishing to pursue careers find they must work at least part-time to meet financial obligations in our increasingly inflationary economy. These women additionally are faced with finding adequate day care and confronting the guilt nearly all working mothers experience.

Furthermore, modern women do not have the sources of emotional support available a generation ago. Their mates often need as much reassurance as they do, and even in suburban towns and cities, expectant couples are unlikely to have friends who are also expecting.

Today's expectant parents are also faced with an immense array of medical choices, precipitated by rapid advances in obstetrical technology. Often decisions are difficult because the possible dangers remain unclear. For example, women over thirty often are advised to undergo amniocentesis, an extraction of fluid from the uterus used to determine possible fetal defects. Parents then have the choice of terminating or continuing the pregnancy. One possible side effect of amniocentesis, however, is spontaneous abortion or miscarriage. While this risk is slight, many women over thirty already have had a difficult time conceiving and dread such a possibility.

Other procedures such as ultrasound (sonograms), fetal monitoring, and the use of certain medications to induce labor have been subject to questions about maternal or fetal health. These concerns add to the mounting list of anxiety-provoking issues likely to affect modern childbearing women.

While tension leads to poor prenatal health, medical research indicates that deep relaxation during labor facilitates an easy, uncomplicated delivery. In his 1987 book, *Mind Over Labor,* childbirth educator Carl Jones cites more than a dozen such studies conducted by medical researchers. He concludes that lovemaking is the only other physical function that is as much affected by emotions as labor. I concur, and would like to add the function of dreaming. The anxiety produced by dreams, particularly nightmares, can have many negative effects, both physiological and psychological. Once you learn to identify and interpret the symbols that cloak your concerns, however, you may even begin to welcome such dreams.

MYTHS AND OLD WIVES' TALES

Women who don't know that dreams represent normal reactions to the very real problems of childbearing naturally become even more anxious and fearful, wondering what such dreams could mean, or if they have some dark significance. Some mothers-to-be have been influenced by old wives' tales, predicting dire outcomes from certain dream elements.

Following are a few of the superstitious interpretations (all of them *false*) ascribed to pregnant women's dreams:

- A dream of a funeral prophesies stillbirth.
- Snakes in third trimester dreams indicate that the umbilical cord is strangling the baby.

- A dream of an ugly or monstrous baby means birth defects.
- Dreams of giving birth to kittens or other small animals indicate that there's something wrong with your baby.
- A dream of your partner with another woman means he's having an affair.
- Dreaming about your former boyfriend or lover suggests that your partner will not be a good father.
- Dreams about your past, especially your teenage years, mean that you are too immature to be a good mother.
- "Barrier" dreams (trying to get over a fence, wall, chasm, and so forth) prophesy a long and difficult labor.

All these "meanings" are pure myths that do not take into account the one important fact established by dream researchers: the interpretation of every dream depends primarily upon very personal associations.

For example, although funerals usually signify the loss of something or someone, pregnant women typically dream of them when they have ended some long-standing habit. Dreams of death and funerals also generally coincide with the withdrawal after cessation of smoking or other addictive behaviors. Therefore, they simply indicate that a "beloved" object (cigarettes) has left one's life forever. In other words, it's quite likely that a funereal dream, even though sad or scary, may actually represent a positive change.

However, even this explanation may not precisely fit your personal associations. Perhaps someone you know or love has been exhibiting symptoms, either subtle or obvious, of declining health. In such a case you might dream of his or her death. Your dreaming self may be sending you this message: you are worried about this person; maybe you should inquire about his or her health. Or you may associate a funereal dream with something or someone in your life that you'd be better off without. Your dreaming self may be pointing this out to you.

Snakes, kittens, and other animals usually symbolize the fetus in pregnant women's dreams. While dreams of a snake might very well represent the umbilical cord—provided the dreamer thinks of a serpent as something coiled or long and tubular—it rarely, if ever, indicates more than that. It does not mean that the baby is in danger of strangulation. Similarly, other animal symbols do not infer an unhealthy fetus. On the contrary, since most women think of kittens and other small animals as adorable, dreams of these cuddly creatures probably indicate your growing love for the unborn child.

The same logic applies to dreams about your partner's infidelity, your own former lovers, and your past generally. These visions usually reflect *anxieties* about losing your mate, rather than the actuality or likelihood of such an event taking place.

So-called "barrier" dreams similarly express fear of labor. Also, it's wise to remember that each individual associates dream elements differently. For example, one volunteer dreamed her husband stood behind a barrier she could not cross. In this case, the wall represented the woman's fear that her husband might not be there when she needed him.

As you read this book, you will learn how to interpret the bizarre symbols of your dreams in a less frightening manner. Then you can identify the personal sources of anxiety triggering these strange dreams.

THE SIX MAJOR FEARS DURING PREGNANCY

My research indicates that there are six major causes of anxiety experienced by today's pregnant women. These typically fall into the following categories:

- Fear that your baby will be deformed or die
- Fear of being an inadequate parent

- Fear of losing your mate
- Fear of a difficult delivery
- Fear of loss of control over your body and emotions
- Fear of financial burdens

Women who are intelligent, well-read, and enlightened appear to be just as prone to these worries as those from a lower economic status or educational level. In fact, the college graduates and successful career women I studied displayed a somewhat higher level of anxiety about these issues, possibly because of their tendency to repress negative emotions or their reluctance to admit to any insecurities about their demanding life-styles.

The fact that educated women may be more aware of the possible side effects of new obstetrical technology also may account in part for their anxiety. Additionally, these expectant mothers tend to be older than those who don't work outside the home, so they have a bit more foundation for normal concerns about complicated deliveries or unhealthy babies. These explanations may also account for the fact that the women I've studied who have already had children (multiparae) suffer from one or more of these fears.

Whatever the reasons, the six major sources of anxiety appear to be no respecters of age or background. Participants in my doctoral study ranged in age from eighteen to thirty-five and claimed a wide variety of educational and economic levels, yet their dreams consistently reflected similar concerns. The following excerpts illustrate the typical fear that the baby may be deformed or die:

> *Alicia, a 32-year-old journalist:* The doctors looked doubtful . . . told me it (the newborn) might not live . . . Then she flopped over and died.

> *Sandra, 34-year-old homemaker, multipara:* My stomach became transparent and I saw a baby with only one arm and a harelip.

Lucie, 18-year-old supermarket checker: There, sitting between my legs, was this naked little boy . . . his face was like an old man's and there were fangs coming out of his lips.

All these women delivered normal, healthy babies, as did most of the others who reported similar dreams. However, many of them underwent needless anxiety; those who suffered from severe tension and stress also had long and sometimes complicated labors.

Mothers-to-be probably always have worried that their unborn might not be healthy. However, dreams reflecting this fear may be more common today than ever before, because of media coverage about the dangers older pregnant women face, such as Down's syndrome and other birth defects.

In *Having a Baby After 30,* the Lamaze authority Elizabeth Bing and Dr. Libby Colman cite studies on maternal age and birth malformations. They point out that, while there exists a slightly higher risk for the babies of older mothers, the majority of these problems occur in women over forty. Even if a forty-plus parent miscarries or decides to terminate the pregnancy after amniocentesis, it is quite probable that the next fetus will grow into a normal, healthy child. Genetic counselors can help women over forty decide on these risks.

For most other expectant mothers under forty, nightmares about a defective fetus have little basis in fact. Rather, they mirror the normal worries that this book seeks to dispel.

Fears of being an inadequate parent also have plagued expectant mothers for generations. Again, these concerns appear to be more prevalent for contemporary pregnant women. Many new mothers today come from smaller families and have not cared for infant sisters and brothers. Older expectant parents also may feel less optimism and energy than they did during their teens and twenties. However, even couples over thirty can take heart from the fact that eighteen- and twenty-year-olds have these nightmares.

Moreover, women who already have children are equally concerned about their parental ability. Some typical dreams include

> *Sheila, 23-year-old legal secretary:* Our apartment was invaded with mice, lizards, rabbits, kittens, puppies. They were coming in the windows and front door. I couldn't stop them and they were messing up everything.

> *Marie, 19-year-old receptionist:* Instead of adults, all the people who came to our office were little kids. They climbed onto my desk, broke my phones, and made a lot of noise. I began to panic and called the police.

> *Francine, 33-year-old homemaker, multipara, pregnant with twins:* Someone left a box full of baby chicks on our doorstep. I was busy with my small son and they died before I had time to take care of them.

Sheila's dream of the small, uncontrollable animals (symbolizing her unborn child), and Marie's nightmare of being invaded by wild youngsters both reflect typical anxiety about being an inadequate parent. An only child, Sheila told me, "I never took care of anything small, not even pets. My folks had two German Shepherds, but Dad always bathed and trained them. In my teens, when other girls my age were baby-sitting, I was tutoring bigger kids in math and chemistry. I don't know if I'll be able to take care of a tiny, helpless baby."

In Lamaze classes, Sheila and her husband received basic instructions on care of the newborn. Marie's hospital maternity nurses helped her learn to diaper and feed her healthy baby boy.

Francine's worry that she might not be able to mother three small children manifested itself in her dream about the dying baby chicks (symbolic of the twin fetuses she was carrying). This fear also is typical of multiparae who expect only one additional baby. It's quite natural that a mother's love for the child or children she's already had may cause her to wonder how she will manage and avoid making the older ones feel neglected or jealous. However, this very sensitivity to her family's needs will often be enough to help her minimize sibling rivalry.

If you are expecting another child, this book suggests ways to cope. Francine gave birth to two identical little girls, and her toddler was allowed to visit her and the new babies immediately afterward. A support group for parents of twins also aided Francine and her husband in effectively dealing with their small son's jealousy of the infants.

Although most studies of pregnant women's dreams have shown that the most frequent character other than self was one's mother, my investigation revealed that the husband now occupies this position. Usually, he simply happens to be there, rather than as a major element in a conflict the dreamer is trying to resolve. However, thirty-two percent of the dreams containing references to husbands did reflect concern about the marital relationship or fear that the mate would be lost through death or some other catastrophe. For example:

> *Eve, 28-year-old cashier:* Saw my husband standing behind this barrier . . . tried to jump over it but couldn't because of the baby. When I woke up, had to wake him just to be sure he was really alive.

> *Faith, 29-year-old nurse:* Out the porthole I saw Joe being blown apart.

> *Belinda, 31-year-old homemaker, wife of an Air Force officer:* Several planes crashed . . . tried to drag (husband) out but he was tangled up in his burning chute . . . I began to cry. There was nothing I could do.

> *Jean, 26-year-old aerobics teacher:* I came home early and saw a woman driving off. In the house, I could smell her perfume and her hairpins were scattered on the bed pillows.

Eve's fear of losing her mate was exaggerated by concerns about his health. His father had died of a heart attack, and

Eve's own father had died when she was a child. Even though her husband had been pronounced healthy by both a cardiologist and the family physician, her dreams continued to reveal persistent anxiety.

In 1978 Dr. Judith Ballou described the pregnant woman's increasing dependence upon her husband and fears that he may not meet her needs. Both Faith and Belinda experienced numerous nightmares about these issues. While Belinda's worries were more realistic (since her pilot husband engaged in somewhat dangerous work), Faith's husband Joe was a civilian in good health, who was unlikely to encounter any perilous conditions.

When we discussed her nightmare, Faith noticed that "blown apart"—the phrase she used to describe Joe's disaster—really meshed with her feelings about how he would react in the delivery room. "I'm a nurse and used to seeing blood and pain," she explained, "but Joe's not. I'm going to need his coaching and I guess I'm afraid he'll just be blown apart by it all."

Fear of loss of the mate to another woman is also a prevalent source of anxiety. As the pregnant woman's waistline expands, so does this concern. Few expectant mothers seem to realize how beautiful (and yes, even sexy!) they are becoming.

With the discomforts of morning sickness and hormonal imbalance behind them, most pregnant women's complexions take on a special, radiant glow. Yet when they look in the mirror, all they see is their bulging tummies and enlarged breasts; they wonder how their mates could possibly find them attractive. Women like Jean, who have been athletic or seriously involved in fitness programs, may experience intense fear as their bodies change. When I lectured at a convention of the International Childbirth Educators Association, several instructors told me of their concerns about pregnant women who literally starve themselves to remain slim.

In the past, obstetricians have advised expectant mothers to restrict calorie intake and avoid salt. Dr. Thomas Brewer, a renowned expert on pregnancy nutrition, now strongly urges pregnant women to avoid low-calorie, low-salt diets that fail to provide enough protein for either the mother or the growing fetus. He suggests a goal of 2,600 calories and 100 grams of protein per day for the average pregnant woman. Adherence to Brewer's carefully balanced diet plan will not keep you skinny during your pregnancy. What it will do is assure that your baby won't have a lower than normal birth weight and that you will be getting all the protein, iron, and vitamins you both need.

Several pregnant women have asked me, "Since I cannot remain healthy without getting a huge belly, what *can* I do to keep my man interested?" This book teaches you how to release the nagging worry that your partner may find you less appealing, or even have an affair. By sharing these concerns with your mate and using your dreams and fantasies to create a new attitude about your body image, you will deepen his intimacy and love.

Interestingly, expectant fathers also dream that their wives are being unfaithful. Such dreams usually arise because impending parenthood brings with it an awareness of changes, that life-styles soon will be quite different and may cause our partners to view us accordingly.

Most women who unconsciously fear their mates' lack of emotional support also have nightmares about difficult deliveries. These are excerpts from typical dreams:

Julia, 33-year-old dental hygienist: Dreamt I was in biology class . . . having to dissect this frog. My partner stuck a piece of cotton with chloroform on it in my face. I woke up with a sickening smell in my nose.

Beverly, 27-year-old homemaker: The doctor comes into the labor room and I am screaming and thrashing about . . . He leaves me to have the baby alone.

Eve (who dreamed of her husband behind a barrier, above): I was at . . . a rocky beach . . . a lot of rocks, slanted with water rushing . . . saw crocodiles in the water.

Anna, 30-year-old office manager: I had the baby on the way to the hospital without any help from the doctor . . . Everything in the car was a mess . . . We were frantically looking for some string to tie the cord.

Both Julia's and Beverly's nightmares reflected their fears of a difficult delivery. However, Julia remained determined not to be sedated during labor, whereas Beverly was almost obsessed with the idea that she would never get through it without epidural anesthesia. Julia also feared that obstetrical personnel might force her to be drugged (represented in her dream by the chloroform). Conversely, Beverly's dream doctor left her alone, without relief, to bear her child. Her husband was not there to give support, either.

Eve's nightmare of climbing over a rocky chasm where rushing tides and crocodiles awaited is quite typical of late pregnancy dreams. The turbulent water (symbolizing labor), the large, menacing animals (depicting emergence of the baby), and the generally vivid details are common traits as the dreamer nears delivery.

Anna's dream of giving birth on the way to the hospital also represents a typical fear that delivery will be a grueling, chaotic experience. While rarely painless or easy, childbirth comes most easily to women who are confident, relaxed, and looking forward to the miraculous occasion.

With six months or more of tension and confusion behind her, however, the laboring woman may not greet delivery with such an exemplary attitude. As one expectant mother in her second month commented, "If I'm out of control now, how will I ever be able to get hold of myself when the contractions actually begin?"

A fear of unchecked emotions and body functions is the fifth major source of anxiety for most pregnant women. Some of this fear has its roots in the unpredictable hormonal activities and resulting mood swings of early pregnancy. Or expectant mothers may be subject to unaccountable fits of temper and irritability. These fears and feelings surface in early pregnancy dreams:

> *Charlotte, 35-year-old legal secretary:* Being impatient with standing in line at the supermarket, I started throwing cans and boxes at the people ahead of me. I'd never do that in real life!

> *Patty, 24-year-old homemaker:* At a shopping mall, saw some guys I knew from high school . . . beat them up pretty badly.

> *Lauren, 32-year-old kindergarten teacher:* Dreamed I was on the playground in the rain. I was crying so hard the children got scared . . . woke up sobbing for no apparent reason.

As the pregnancy progresses, some women continue to worry about this loss of control, even though they superficially appear to be on a more even emotional keel. For instance, the following expectant moms claimed they had no such fears; their dreams indicated otherwise:

> *Sue, 27-year-old advertising copywriter:* Dreamt my car was out of control, speeding down a steep hill. Suddenly my legs were paralyzed . . . couldn't do anything to stop . . . woke up when I crashed.

> *Pauline, 33-year-old bank teller:* I was on a sailboat when our pet collie dog jumped on board . . . he leaped onto me, making me let go of the lines . . . my labor started . . . we capsized . . . couldn't swim and kept going under. (Actually I'm a very good swimmer.)

> *Doreen, 21-year-old waitress:* Tried to help this old lady sit down but I tripped and fell, knocking her over . . . the whole building fell down in a sudden earthquake.

Nightmares featuring out-of-control vehicles are reported by people who are not pregnant, especially when confronted with life's circumstances that seem beyond their reach. However, such dreams happen frequently—with somewhat different themes—to expectant women. Sue's inability to control her speeding car was further complicated by her sudden paralysis. Similar dreams also may include elements of "being invaded." The accident caused by a leaping dog (representing the third trimester fetus) provides an example.

The feeling of one's body (Pauline's sailboat) being exposed to invasion is natural, and no cause for guilt. Such dreams merely portray a realization that another human has indeed captured a very private part of you. Surprise and fear are normal reactions.

More than forty years ago, Dr. Helene Deutsch noted that most pregnant women have such feelings and that these usually subside after the expectant mother has "incorporated" her baby mentally and emotionally. However, modern women appear to find this gradual, yet ever-increasing, lack of body control more upsetting than they did in Deutsch's time. Accustomed to being self-sufficient and independent, they do not like relying on their mates and others to do the small tasks that their enlarging abdomens and general clumsiness make difficult for them. Therefore, Doreen's nightmare of being unable to help an old lady— and even of crashing to the ground like an earthquake-shattered building—is hardly surprising.

Independence probably remains one of the underlying reasons for the sixth major source of anxiety contemporary pregnant women undergo: the fear of financial burdens. A continuing rise in the cost of living concerns most expectant couples. Even women who have successful careers and adequate health insurance worry about increasing medical fees, day care, and the possible loss of income should they be unable to work after childbirth.

Many unemployed new mothers are forced to take part- or full-time jobs to help make ends meet. Those who have become accustomed to a few luxuries may resent cutbacks or may worry about the dwindling possibility of affording their own home. Naturally, many pregnant women's dreams relate to these concerns:

Albertine, 33-year-old photographer: Dreamed I was in labor . . . refused admittance to the hospital because our credit was bad . . . had the baby on the sidewalk.

Debby, 26-year-old homemaker: Waiting in line at the cashier's in a department store . . . no money in my wallet! So I put the layette things in my shopping bag and left. I stole those things! Woke up feeling scared and guilty.

Annie, 30-year-old secretary: A terrible war was on . . . the baby, my husband, and I were living in a shack made of cardboard boxes.

While there is no magical way to obtain overnight wealth, this book provides a number of approaches for realistic financial management and suggestions to relieve worries about economic burdens.

Once you generally begin to understand the meaning of your bizarre and often nightmarish dreams, you will learn how to work with them and the anxieties they represent. Pregnant women who followed the easy instructions in the upcoming chapters discovered that their nightmares were replaced with new, positive, and healing dreams.

The Five-Step Program

To help you achieve relaxation and freedom from anxiety, this book provides a simple, five-step program for comprehending dreams and other states of consciousness during pregnancy. As I outlined in the Introduction, these techniques involve

- Keeping a dream diary
- Understanding dream symbols and diagramming your dreams
- Understanding your emotions
- Interpreting your dreams
- Controlling your dreams

THE DREAM DIARY

Often, pregnant women begin to write down their dreams, even if they haven't done so before conception. Many tell me that they were so struck by the unusual qualities of their sleeping visions that they tried to capture them on paper. If you already are recording your dreams, you may have discovered that it's rarely easy to translate them into words. An understanding of their origins and connections with your waking life will render this task less frustrating.

You may want to start your dream diary by purchasing a looseleaf notebook with an attractive cover. This type will be the easiest to use, since you can scatter extra pages in convenient locations: your bathroom, the kitchen, or the other places you usually go when you wake up during the night.

Once you've chosen your blank book, make daily entries, including your dreams and brief notes about any negative thoughts you may have had. Describing those negative attitudes helps you to learn methods of changing them into more positive ones. This exercise ultimately adds to your growing arsenal of anxiety-defeating skills.

The section on creating your dream diary also gives you tips on recall, capturing elusive details, and remembering your subconscious feelings before they're forgotten.

As you continue reading this book, you will want to include other entries—dream diagrams, notes about your dream levels and patterns, and records of creative daydreams or fantasies.

DREAM SYMBOLS, DREAM DIAGRAMS

Please don't be intimidated by these academic-sounding terms! A dream symbol merely means an object or character representing something in your waking life. For instance, when pregnant women dream about small animals, these usually symbolize the fetus.

However, it's always important to bear in mind that your personal association to any dream element provides the best clue to its true meaning. Try on a typical meaning the way you might a hat or dress—if it doesn't fit, don't buy it.

Most pregnant women have similar physical and emotional experiences, and the symbols in their dreams are usually comparable. The majority of women in labor liken the ebb and flow of ocean tides to contractions, yet there are always exceptions.

Jane, a 34-year-old homemaker, was in her third trimester when she dreamed that her twelve-year-old son Bobby was swept out to sea in a storm. Jane thought this dream related to her concern about Bobby's important math exam the next day. Before retiring, Jane had coached Bobby and noticed how worried he was about the test, since he wouldn't be allowed to remain on the soccer team if he failed. Diverging from the pregnancy norm, this multiparous mom also claimed her previous contractions in no way reminded her of ocean waves.

You can identify dream symbols by noting the principal nouns (such as characters or objects) in your dream record. Circle each one and then jot down your associations to them. To help clarify the action or plot of your dream, also underline the major verbs or action words. This circling and underlining is all you need to "diagram" your dreams. Although some psychologists teach other, more complicated methods, this simple system usually suffices in helping my students begin to grasp the meaning of their dreams. The chapter on recording and diagramming dreams provides more detailed directions for this easy procedure.

EMOTIONS

One of the most important clues to your dream's meaning is the way you feel both during and immediately after it. My experience suggests that most people don't know how to describe or even identify their emotions. When I show concern about a client whose attitude appears hostile and whose entire body language seems to exude anger, the reply is frequently, "Oh, I'm feeling okay, maybe a little annoyed." Pregnant women often become more introverted than before, so their tendency to be noncommunicative about their emotions increases.

When I interviewed expectant mothers regarding their nightmares, many failed to recall how they felt during the dream, even though gruesome events were taking place; however, most remembered feeling frightened upon awakening. The same lack of awareness characterized descriptions of obviously sad, painful, or even happy dreams. The women often used vague terms such as "nervous," "frustrated" "upset," "bad," or "nice."

While it is always a good idea to be able to identify your feelings, comprehending your emotions is of utmost importance during pregnancy. If you're not aware that you're feeling tense because you're scared or angry, it's difficult to learn how to express or release these emotions. Chapter 5 provides guidelines for the identification of feelings, explains the physical changes accompanying each emotion, and examines the dreams that depict them.

INTERPRETING YOUR DREAMS

After mastering the first three steps described above, you will find it easy to translate the messages your inner self is sending. The next portion of the book will explain some of the finer points of interpretation, including dream levels, patterns, and rare and unusual dreams.

Although your first reaction to your dream symbols is generally correct, as your interpretive skills improve you will find that most of your dreams have more than one explanation or level of meaning. For example, Jane's dream of her twelve-year-old being swept out to sea also could have meant that she was concerned about the effect the new baby might have on him.

As we discussed her initial interpretation and talked about Bobby's recent difficulties with math, it occurred to Jane that her unexpected pregnancy already could be making her son feel somewhat pushed aside. Jane commented, "Maybe my dream was telling me that Bobby is feeling swept away by his Dad's and my preoccupation with this pregnancy."

When we further reviewed Jane's records, we discovered three other dreams revolving around her son's schoolwork. "His teacher asked me just last month if everything was okay at home," Jane remembered, "and I said there was nothing different or special going on. Can't believe I said that!"

CONTROLLING YOUR DREAMS

My pregnant students also have learned to control and work with their dreams much more rapidly than nonpregnant people in other workshops. The techniques they use include "dream incubation" and "lucid dreaming."

Although the term "dream incubation" has been employed for a number of years by psychologists who work with clients of both sexes, it seems especially appropriate for the pregnant woman. An incubated dream is one that you decide to have before falling asleep. Although it sounds difficult, this technique is merely a further refinement of recall. You must become deeply relaxed and then silently give your inner self directions about the topic you wish to dream. Although you may have to practice several nights before achieving results, you—like most of the pregnant women I've taught—will soon be able to focus on your baby or any other subject you choose.

Dr. Stephen LaBerge, author of *Lucid Dreaming,* defines this phenomenon as a heightened, almost awake awareness encountered *during the dream.* Although most people awaken then, it is possible to learn how to have a lucid dream and remain asleep. Much more difficult to achieve than dream incubation, my adaptation of LaBerge's technique also proved successful for a number of pregnant women.

I'm convinced that one of the reasons expectant mothers master both of these unusual dream states so much more easily than other people is that they almost always find themselves in an altered state of consciousness, somewhat similar to a light trance. Again, I have no statistics, nor have I conducted investigations which might provide data for this hypothesis. However, my assumption is based on observations of hundreds of pregnant women, the majority of whom appear to possess these characteristics.

Pregnant Women's Unusual Waking States

As a group, pregnant women have a number of waking personality traits that distinguish them from others. These include the tendency to be moody, absentminded, dreamy, and drowsy; the tendency to fantasize and daydream; self-preoccupation; and phobias.

Even before you begin to "show," you probably will develop the extreme mood swings we've already discussed. Sometimes these unpredictable, see-saw feelings persist into late pregnancy, although they usually subside by the fourth month.

From time to time, you also will notice that you're absentminded, misplacing keys or shopping lists or forgetting important appointments. On social occasions you may find yourself drifting off into a dreamy, euphoric state while others engage in animated conversation. Jackie, a 35-year-old journalist expecting her third child, told me, "It's embarrassing sometimes. The other day I almost fell asleep during our own dinner party!"

Jackie also admitted that she showed a tendency to fantasize and daydream in a distressingly realistic manner. "Several times," she confided, "I've had experiences which were like dreams, except that I'm sure I was awake. At first, I thought I was going crazy." Fortunately, Jackie's husband and several friends were familiar with what psychologists call "altered states of consciousness," and they were able to reassure her.

Jackie's preoccupation with her moods and feelings typifies the self-preoccupation characteristic of most pregnant women. This does not imply egotism or selfishness. Rather, it is a natural reaction to the increasing vulnerability that both mother and unborn child endure as the pregnancy progresses. Feeling clumsy and unprotected, the expectant woman may spend much energy and thought trying to withdraw from possible harm. Dr. Helene Deutsch initially commented on this trait in 1945. It was again noted by Dr. G. Bibring in 1959, Dr. Terese Benedek in 1970, and by Drs. Libby and Arthur Colman in 1972. The news is that contemporary pregnant women falsely view this turning inward as yet another symptom of the onset of abnormal behavior.

Expectant mothers who develop phobias for the first time also become alarmed. For instance, Sue suddenly became phobic about driving her car. Carolyn, whose office was on an upper floor of a tall building, felt dizzy when she looked out the window. Such phobias arise suddenly and seem to disappear after the baby is born. In addition, many women who have them also describe other, more unusual altered states, such as Jackie's hallucinatory type daydreams.

If you're an expectant mother subject to these unusual experiences, you needn't worry: more pregnant women share them than most obstetrical professionals suspect. A lot of moms-to-be refuse to discuss the issue with their physicians, fearing ridicule, embarrassment, or being judged mentally abnormal.

Psychologist Dr. Ronald K. Siegel, a professor of psychopharmacology at UCLA, says that Altered States of Consciousness (ASCs) evoke another mode of thinking, feeling, and perceiving—much like intoxication. While these experiences can be induced by something as mild as daydreams or as traumatic as a near-death experience, in nonpregnant patients they're commonly thought to be symptoms of a pathological nature or of a drug-induced state.

When expectant mothers have them, the likely explanation differs. Two major factors seem to be at work behind pregnant women's ASCs: physiological changes and transitions of life-crisis proportions.

Just as these two theories both apply to expectant mothers' dreams, so they may help explain their decidedly different waking state. There's no doubt that sudden hormonal changes, such as increased progesterone and estrogen, affect all emotions, perceptions, and reactions to other people and events.

Higher levels of progesterone are necessary because they help the embryo attach to the uterine lining. At the same time, this increase can have a depressing effect on the central nervous system, imitating a premenstrual symptom. Tracy Hotchner, a highly respected childbirth researcher and journalist, also indicates that rapid rises in progesterone and estrogen levels may precipitate a dazed feeling. Light trance states indeed are typical of ASCs.

Feelings of disorientation, often described at OBEs, or out-of-body experiences, also prove to be common stress symptoms. In an article on hallucinations for the December 1988 issue of *OMNI,* Dr. Siegel describes a patient whose tests showed both high blood pressure and severe stress. This man remained convinced that his mind was being controlled by a machine. Since tension and stress are often the precursors of hallucinations in nonpregnant people, it's not surprising that expectant mothers should go through the same sensations.

The next chapter, devoted entirely to the anatomy of consciousness, provides more detailed descriptions of the ways your mind and brain operate in connection with all these internal and external stimuli. Later, you will learn how altered states may be employed to enhance deep relaxation and cope with the normal anxieties of pregnancy.

Instead of feeling at the mercy of outside influences, you can be in control and turn these altered states into tools that will give you sweeter, healing dreams and even help you communicate with your unborn child. Your dreams and fantasies come from a wise and loving part of your mind, your inner self.

With this book as a guide, you can penetrate a wonderful, mysterious realm. Learn to use inner knowledge to enhance your pregnancy and your relationship. The resulting emotional growth will not only show you where you've been and where you're going but should also provide both you and your mate with the skills needed for future parenthood.

CHAPTER 2

Where Do Dreams Come From?

Dreams, daydreams, and fantasies do not originate in our brains; these experiences partially reflect the events and interactions that occur with others during our waking lives. These stimuli come from our various senses and are then processed and stored in the brain. When we sleep, some of this information surfaces.

Brain activity slows down in the initial stage of sleep, as do many other body functions, including breathing, heartbeat, and temperature. After a period of deep and restful relaxation, these functions gradually accelerate. Next, certain neurons are fired from the brain stem. We "see" fantastic colors and images, and begin to dream. Another area of the brain brings to our attention previous reactions to similar stimuli, weaving a story from the pictures being projected onto the mind's eye.

Still other brain systems are at work when we experience daydreams and fantasies. To better understand these intricate processes, it helps to have a general knowledge of the shape and functions of the brain, from which arises *consciousness.*

The Anatomy of Consciousness

Think of your brain as an organic computer—similar to a large, three-pound greyish walnut. Different areas of this complex structure control specific activities: sensations, feelings and emotions, images and pictures, and thoughts and ideas. This entire mental process makes up your consciousness and begins before birth. When the fetus is only six months old, its brain already receives, processes, and stores a multitude of sensations occurring even in its small, safe uterine environment. The unborn child cannot see, but it reacts appropriately to movement, touch, and sound. Evidence of these reactions has been found by a number of prenatal researchers, including Albert Liley, Erik Wedenberg, and Bjorn Johannson. In *Emotion: A Psychoevolutionary System,* Dr. Robert Plutchik describes the theory that, when the brain receives stimuli, it both stores the information and records the resulting feelings and emotions.

Thus, the fetus has certain body sensations that become associated with pleasure, pain, fear, or other feelings. Sudden movement, loud noises, being pricked or pinched may cause discomfort so that forever afterward the child will relate them to pain. The emotion of fear then becomes attached in our minds with the event that previously made us uncomfortable. Conversely, mother's heartbeat, parents' voices, and soothing music become associated with pleasure to such an extent that these sounds will often quiet a cranky newborn.

With the added sensations of sight and smell after birth, the brain receives much more information but processes it in a similar fashion. Thus, we quickly learn to anticipate pleasurable body feelings when we smell or see something associated with comfort and nurturance. We later may only need to recall an image to sense pleasure or pain.

Connected by intricate nerve nets and special cells, many areas of the brain interact to perform these tasks. The brain also simultaneously monitors every organ in the complex body. What follows is a brief, simplified explanation of these extremely intricate processes.

FUNCTIONS OF THE BRAIN

For purposes of understanding dreams and other states of consciousness arising during pregnancy, one only needs to know general brain functions. According to the Russian neuropsychologist A. R. Luria, these are

- Regulating tone or waking
- Obtaining, processing, and storing information
- Programming, regulating, and verifying mental activity

Dr. Luria explains that each of these sections of the brain is interconnected. Therefore, it's difficult for the lay person to understand that the precise site of each unit cannot be pinpointed on a standard, textbook drawing. The unit regulating "tone," the level of alertness in the brain's cortical area, is located mainly in the brain stem. It, too, boasts a complex network of nerves that affect all other brain areas, allowing us to be awake and attentive when the need arises.

The brain unit receiving, processing, and storing information mainly does its work in the neocortex, near the back of the head on the surface of the brain's two hemispheres. This unit differs from the one that regulates tone because it consists of isolated cells called neurons. These neurons "fire" or send off specific signals, causing us to see, hear, smell, taste, and feel.

The third brain unit, perhaps the most complex of all, is located in the frontal regions of the brain, at the top of the head just above the forehead. This component has the formidable task of examining incoming information and then programming it to direct and regulate specific behavior. While monitoring our actions and providing feedback, the unit also helps us decide whether to verify results or make appropriate changes.

Just as a computer could not operate efficiently without intricate circuitry and connectors, so the complex areas of our brains depend upon one another to function properly. It is very important to understand this interaction because many people get the impression that the two sides, or hemispheres, of our brains operate independently.

RIGHT BRAIN, LEFT BRAIN

The two halves of our brains work in different styles, but they both contribute to much of our waking mental activity and are physically connected by a bridge of brain tissue called the *corpus callosum.* Interestingly, recent research shows that the callosum in women's brains is usually larger and stronger than in men's. Because this connecting tissue lets one hemisphere know what the other does, females also seem to be better able to recall dreams. Finally, this may help account for the fact that most women are more consciously aware of their emotions.

Even though the two hemispheres of the brain connect, one side usually remains dominant, or more active and efficient, than the other. In general, the left side prevails in people with mathematical skills and a logical tendency. Those who possess dominant right hemispheres are more likely to be creative and intuitive. They tend to grasp the entire meaning of a situation rather than understanding or being able to analyze its parts.

Members of either gender can have left- or right-brain thinking styles. Even those who claim left-brain personalities, however, go through developmental stages when the right hemisphere appears to be stronger, and vice versa. Pregnancy is one of those times when the right brain becomes enhanced in women. Increased levels of estrogen and progesterone probably contribute to this phenomenon. It also seems fitting for the expectant mother to be especially preoccupied with such right-brain thoughts as creativity and nurturing.

Until recently, sleep researchers thought that dreams

arose from the right hemisphere. Their reasoning proved understandable: while the left brain rests—in sleep or during deep, trancelike relaxation—the right hemisphere presents us with images and pictures from a vast storehouse of memories, past and present. However, Dr. John Antrobus, a psychologist at the City University of New York, observed that *both* hemispheres remain active during sleep. Current research now indicates that dreams probably arise from another type of brain activity.

THE BRAIN CHEMISTRY OF DREAMS

According to the new theory, dream images begin in the brain stem. This section actually represents a continuation of the spinal cord. As the "stalk" emerges from the spine, it thickens and spreads into the upper regions of the brain. Neuroscientists Robert W. McCauley and J. Allan Hobson of Harvard Medical School now believe that the brain stem emits impulses at the end of the deeply restful stage of sleep. A series of neurons is then fired off.

This activity floods the brain with a chemical substance called *acetylcholine,* a neurotransmitter used to signal other nerve cells. When this substance is active, other brain cells which use different kinds of transmitters are subdued. Acetylcholine also stimulates visual images.

This theory explains the fact that a dreamer's eyelids begin to twitch rapidly (called Rapid Eye Movement or REM sleep) even though most of the body remains inert. When we're awake, visual signals cause movements, such as walking, running, and other physical activity. Although the brain may desire activity during sleep, it gets no response because the acetylcholine shuts off the nerve links that signal motion.

The frontal part of the brain, described by Dr. Luria as being responsible for examining and programming incoming information, is now confronted with messages indicating activity—even though the dreamer's body remains inert.

Trying to make sense of its own internal signals, the sleeping brain dips into its storehouse of memories, gives meaning to images, and weaves a story to explain them. In a recent article on dreaming, Dr. Hobson suggests that each person's dream visions may contain elements that reflect issues unique to him or her. Thus, the action or plot of the dream story almost always connects with something in our waking life: a personal attitude or belief system, an unresolved or ignored conflict, or perhaps a secret wish or fantasy.

When the frontal brain receives images via neurons fired from the brain stem, the right brain probably plays an active part in processing images. Because this hemisphere "thinks" in pictures rather than words or logical thoughts, it may make more sense of the randomly fired colors and shapes than the left brain. An understanding of the traits of both hemispheres also makes it easier to interpret dreams and other altered states of consciousness.

THE HEMISPHERIC MODEL OF DREAM INTERPRETATION

Bear in mind that the left hemisphere controls most of our language skills and that the right hemisphere thinks in images and pictures. Once you have learned to translate pictures into words, you'll be well on the way toward interpreting your dreams.

For example, when Jane dreamed that her twelve-year-old son Bobby was "swept out to sea," she probably envisioned images and colors resembling a small figure surrounded by high waves. Later, as her waking, left brain tried to understand this dream, Jane realized that she perceived her son as being swept away by the events surrounding her unexpected pregnancy.

Once we understand the traits of right- and left-brain activity, it becomes easier to comprehend why many dreams seem to be so unreal or illogical upon rising. The left brain begins to take over when we are half-awake, analyzing everything and trying to make sense of it. This hemisphere also controls most of our language skills. So when it is confronted with a memory of moving, three-dimensional pictures, it desperately attempts to put all the pieces together in an order corresponding to our perceived waking lives.

Usually, your waking mind will think, "This is nonsense! Nothing like what I dreamed could happen in real life!" However, if we give the left brain a bit more time to translate the pictures into words, we begin to make sense of those weird dreams. This translation is what psychologists refer to as "dream symbols." Later chapters will teach you an easy way to unravel the meaning of the symbols that fill your own dreams during pregnancy.

DREAMLIKE STATES

Expectant mothers can even experience other dreamlike states while they're awake, including daydreams and fantasies, visions, and premonitions.

What triggers daydreams and fantasies is another unsolved mystery. Dr. Jerome L. Singer of Yale University, a pioneer in modern daydream research, and Dr. Antrobus developed a questionnaire which has since been used by dozens of other psychologists in their efforts to explain these types of waking mental activities. While we still do not understand the precise reasons for daydreams and fantasies, various studies suggest that they pop into our consciousness when we happen upon a "cue," relating to some current problem or concern.

For example, in her first pregnancy with twins, Jackie imagined that one of them magically came out of her abdomen, took her hand, and flew around the room with her. The cue for this daydream might have been the "quickening"— the first noticeable movement of fetal life—Jackie felt just before this ASC occurred.

Additionally, daydreams happen most often when we're doing something that does not require our full attention.

Our minds then move on to a current concern in need of resolution. Since the left brain is usually involved with the task at hand, the right brain emits a kind of movie or waking dream, similar in structure to a sleeping dream. Visions, on the other hand, seem more realistic than daydreams because the person who experiences them believes the events actually take place, at least until the experience ends. Visions are commonly associated with hallucinogenic drugs, hypnosis, meditation and profoundly religious states, and certain mental disorders such as schizophrenia. If you're pregnant and subject to occasional visionary experiences, don't be alarmed. As with dreams, the rapidly changing hormone levels in your body may trigger these waking episodes.

Premonitions and intense flashes of intuitive thought also are reported by many pregnant women. It's doubtful that most of these thoughts have any great significance except that they may be the result of repressed fears. Express and release your concerns, rather than ignore them.

Fantasies, visions, and premonitions nevertheless prove fearful because women think they are hallucinating or even losing their minds. Again, the left brain will not understand and may send up warning signals—the source of the inner voice that says, "This is crazy!" or "Ignore this, it's all your imagination!" Just as you can improve the quality of your life by comprehending your dreams, so you can also learn to use these waking, visionary states to enhance your pregnancy and ease some of its discomforts.

In *The Creative Edge,* William C. Miller points out that your mind's ability to generate such images may become one of your best problem-solving tools. While most people must spend a considerable amount of time and effort summoning these imagery skills, during pregnancy you have the advantage of being in close touch with them.

PART TWO

❖

Understanding

❖

Your

❖

Dreams

❖

CHAPTER 3

❖

Step 1: Recording Your Dreams and Creating Daydreams

In order to resolve the anxieties that cause so many of your nightmares, you must understand your dreams and other states of consciousness such as daydreams and fantasies. The first step in my five-step program involves two processes: keeping a diary to record your dreams and using your imagination to create the positive images necessary to counteract your nightmares.

Before you can record your dreams, however, you need to be able to remember them. Sometimes the hectic pace of daily life may make you forget even the most vivid of your nocturnal images.

Most of us have had rude awakenings: the alarm going off, the phone ringing, a hungry child or pet begging attention, or a mate unwittingly intruding into the last moments of a dream. With these interruptions, we may be able to recall only a few disconnected images or forget that we had any dreams at all. Louise told this story in her fourth month of pregnancy:

Early one morning, as the bright rays of sunlight touched my face, I snuggled deeper under the covers. I was in that wonderful, half-asleep state, the "twilight zone." It seemed I was lying on something as light as air, yet it supported my warm, relaxed body. Everything was soft and buoyant: my body, my silky gown, the pale blue sky. Here and there, wisps of feathery white vapor seemed to rise lazily from my bed. Then I realized I was actually resting on a cloud. Blissful feelings and thoughts flitted through my mind: "Wish I could stay here in this sweet place forever. And right here beside me, so close and warm, is . . . I think it's a baby! Or maybe a cuddly, furry little puppy. . . ." Then, my husband's voice cut into my reverie with "Louise, honey—where'd you put the toothpaste?" Ouch! Oh no . . . the cloud and the sweetness . . . they're all going away! Then I sat bolt upright, frowning. Grabbed my robe, rushed to the bathroom to help my hubby find the toothpaste. Later, when I tried to recall that wonderful dream, I could only remember a sense of well-being at the end.

If you have interruptions similar to Louise's, you probably need to make some small changes in your life-style. Explain to your partner that you need to awaken naturally, with a few private minutes to review your dreams and memories. You can then let your waking state take over, allowing you to be alert and available for all those morning chores that tend to drive away the fantasies.

Before you learn to interpret your dreams, you must be able to remember them. Many people forget or only dimly recall their dreams because they have gotten into the habit of letting the left-brain waking state take over too quickly. In fact, some people make the transition in such an abrupt, thoroughly automatic fashion that they claim they never dream. The eminent sleep researcher, Dr. Montague Ullman, co-author of *Working with Dreams,* denies this assertion; in fact, we have from three to five dreams every night, occurring at approximately ninety-minute intervals. Our dreams also become longer as the sleep period progresses. Therefore, the dream just before awakening is usually more complex and is the one we remember most easily.

Pregnant women have a decided advantage over other dreamers because they awaken more often. The enlarged uterus creates pressure on the bladder, necessitating bathroom trips every couple of hours. If your baby has begun to move, it may seem this activity really gets started just about the time you're sinking into a deep, peaceful sleep. These factors combine to wake you more frequently, giving you the advantage of being able to recall two or more dreams every night.

Recording Your Dreams

Psychologists have devised a simple method which makes it possible for anyone to remember dreams: write them down immediately upon awakening. Keep a pad and pen on your night table or in another convenient location. Some women place extra blank pages and writing implements in the bathroom as well.

Recording dreams is a two-part process. First, without moving or opening your eyes, try to remember your most recent thoughts, your dreams. Now, sit up slowly, allowing your body to stay in its relaxed, sleepy mode as long as possible. Next, open your eyes, reach for your pad and pen, and write down whatever you recall. After repeating this simple procedure a few times, you probably will find yourself remembering quite well.

Should your dreams still escape you, try this easy exercise: just before falling asleep, silently repeat, "When I wake up, I will remember my dreams." This statement, when practiced in a relaxed state, has the same effect as a posthypnotic suggestion. You will be surprised to find yourself remembering your dreams much more often and in more detail.

KEEPING A DREAM DIARY

Once you have practiced writing down your dreams, you are ready to start recording them in earnest. Keeping a dream diary is useful because it aids dream recall, permits review of previous dreams, provides space for additional thoughts and comments, and becomes a record of your pregnancy.

Instead of jotting down your dreams on scraps of paper, get a notebook or diary for this purpose. Whatever you choose, keep in mind that you are about to begin the creation of a precious keepsake, one you may want to share with your child in later years. Colleen and Carl, a couple who attended my Relaxation in Pregnancy classes, began reading excerpts from Colleen's diary to their daughter on her second birthday. Now, stories of "when I was in Mommy's tummy" are the child's favorites. This fortunate little girl feels she was always wanted; and her parents also say they cherish her anew as they share their very earliest moments together.

Once you've acquired the book you wish to use, write the date at the top of the first page. Every evening and morning from now until your delivery, make a four-part entry in your dream diary, as follows:

1. At bedtime, briefly note any negative thoughts you recall from that day. For example, in her third month Colleen wrote, "I hate the way my waistline is getting thicker." Two months later she wrote, "I felt really jealous when Carl paid attention to other women at a party tonight." Her seventh month evoked, "Had to leave half the groceries for Carl to put away. It makes me feel so frustrated not to be able to do little things like that."

There are several reasons for emptying your mind of negative thoughts at bedtime. In *Living Your Dreams,* psychologist Gayle Delaney advises her clients to begin each entry with notes about the day's events—especially thoughts and feelings—to clear the mind, aid in relaxation, and focus attention on the journals. My students also find this process cathartic, enabling them to drift off to sleep without having to dwell on stressful matters. With practice you'll even begin to pinpoint the areas of anxiety that may be causing needless tension and worry.

2. Select one of these negative thoughts and turn it into a positive statement. For example, Colleen's comment about her thickening waistline became "My baby is growing and making my body more beautiful day by day." After her negative thought about her husband's attention to other women, she wrote, "Carl and I are creating a new life, a family, together. I trust him; he loves and supports me." Finally, she changed the negative attitude about her clumsiness: "My first priority is carrying and nurturing our baby. I can ask for help with other tasks."

After you have become skilled at reversing the day's adverse thoughts, you will learn how to create positive daydreams to help you deal with the six major sources of anxiety. For now, however, your attitude will change simply by noticing your negative thoughts and attempting to convert them into positive ones. You also will find yourself focusing attention on the issues underlying your dreams.

3. Now, write this statement: "I will remember my dreams." Repeat it over and over as you are falling asleep. When you are drifting into slumber, you will enter a semi-hypnotic state, ideal for absorbing gentle suggestions that can be followed during the waking hours.

4. The next morning—or whenever you rise—*stay in the same position and keep your eyes closed a few moments as you try to recall your dream.* Once the dream is firmly in your mind, open your eyes and get up slowly. Then write a description of your dream memories, as described below.

First, tell what happened. Try to put in as many details as possible. For example, the night after she had written her negative thoughts about her thickening waistline, Colleen recorded this dream:

> Our house had suddenly gotten larger. I was amazed. The kitchen was twice as big and the dining room was huge. Our furniture looked lost in so much space. All the walls were painted pink. I called Mom to tell her and she said we should go shopping right away. I felt scared, not knowing how to cope with this.

Colleen's negative thoughts from the previous day lend a valuable clue about the dream's meaning. The expanding house symbolized her growing abdomen. It's also interesting that the walls were pink, and that Colleen gave birth to a girl. Such dream "prophecies" are not always correct. Many women dream of gender-specific symbols, yet the baby turns out to be the opposite sex. The important thing to note, however, is that Colleen's dreaming self clearly presented a message: to end needless anxiety, she should improve her attitudes about her body image.

If you had more than one dream, number each one and write down whatever you recall. Even if you cannot remember the entire dream, a fragment is worth recording. Sometimes a later reading of these snippets will trigger memories of an entire dream, or at least some additional parts of it. For example, the same night Colleen envisioned the enlarging house, she recalled this portion of another dream:

> *Dream #2:* Something about shopping with my Mom . . . she kept picking out things that were too small for me and I got mad . . . the rest is a blur.

Even though she only recalled a little of this dream, Colleen saw that it also reflected worry about her changing figure. Interestingly, both dreams included her mother. Colleen thus realized that she maintained some old, residual conflicts from her teenage years that begged further discussion and, hopefully, resolution.

Note how you felt both during the dream and upon awakening. Remember that subconscious thoughts nearly always mirror your waking concerns. In Colleen's dream of the expanding house, she felt she would not be able to cope. The fragment about shopping with her Mom indicated anger over the clothes that no longer fit. In her waking life, Colleen both hated her changing body and was afraid that she might not be able to control all the changes taking place.

When recording your dreams, also attempt to establish linkages between certain events. Jot down in parentheses anything that reminds you of an earlier thought or occurrence. For example: "In my dream I was swimming in a lake with a small dog paddling along beside me. (He looked like a puppy I had when I was 6 years old.)" or "I dreamed I was trying to eat some food that tasted scorched. (Yesterday I burned our dinner, and even though my husband was nice about it, I went to bed feeling guilty about being so careless.)" This technique of noting "dream associations"—called "latent dream content" by psychologists—will be important when you embark on interpretation.

Don't worry if your dream makes little sense when you're awake. Often the timing may be distorted, so that something you know happened first appears at the end. Or people (including yourself) will do and say things totally out of context. The confusion takes place because our brain stems are sending us bizarre signals while another part of our brain is weaving a story around these "pictures." Write down whatever you recall—no matter how incredible or ridiculous. As you learn to interpret these symbols, they will begin to make sense.

Finally, at some quiet time during the day, re-read last night's entries, paying special attention to the negative thought that you turned into a positive statement. You will probably discover, as Colleen did, that your dreams appear to reflect one or more self-defeating attitudes. Now is the time to use the power of your imagination to change these negative thoughts.

Creating a Daydream

Like most people, you were probably taught that daydreaming is a waste of time. Parents admonish their children from the earliest years to "stop wool-gathering, gazing out the window, stop doing nothing—pay attention, do your homework." The reprimands continue. Psychologists and neuroscientists now tell us, however, that daydreaming enriches life, enhances our problem-solving abilities, and can even improve physical and emotional health.

Over the past twenty years, Drs. Jerome Singer and John Antrobus have been analyzing the data gleaned from their questionnaire—a tool used by hundreds of psychologists to measure the qualities of daydreams. These researchers define a daydream as a spontaneous and fanciful notion, usually apart from your immediate situation. A daydream may focus on ordinary events or reactions, or on outrageous and extreme possibilities. The process often takes place when you are engaged in monotonous or boring tasks, although difficult or painful activities also evoke waking fantasies.

However, you can also deliberately plan a daydream by choosing a topic and "setting the stage" for your imagination to suggest spontaneous alternatives to a problem or conflict. This process, known as "creative daydreaming," involves the following sequence of steps:

- Selecting the negative issue
- Creating a positive statement
- Relaxing deeply
- Imagining a scenario for the positive statement
- Taping or writing the scenario
- Relaxing deeply and integrating the daydream

SELECTING THE NEGATIVE ISSUE

Consider again the case of Colleen, who found herself developing a poor body image as her pregnancy progressed. Like many American women, she took a deserved pride in her looks and fitness. Colleen worked out daily in a local gym before becoming pregnant and carefully avoided fattening foods. Fortunately, her fitness instructor was well informed about safe dietary and exercise routines during pregnancy. Otherwise, Colleen might have reacted as do some other women: determined to hang onto their prepregnancy figures, they neglect to eat the foods necessary for healthy fetal development.

Despite the reassurances of her gym instructor and her doctor, Colleen remained troubled by the negative body image she had acquired as her waistline expanded. She recorded this nightmare during her third month:

> In this dream I was part of a "girlie" show in a carnival. I was backstage watching the others go out and wriggle around in hula costumes. The barker was yelling out each woman's name as she approached the footlights. "Here comes Wanda! Woo woo!" he yelled, and then Wanda went down into the audience. Then it was my turn. "And now, here's Colleen. Just look at those curves!" I danced out into the spotlight and everyone began laughing and jeering. My husband Carl was sitting in the front row with his arm around Wanda! I looked down at myself and saw that I had this enormous belly sticking out. And my arms and legs had flabby rolls of fat on them. Some men in the audience began booing and yelling, "We didn't come to see the Fat Lady!" I was so embarrassed and then I woke up, feeling awful and wondering if Carl was having an affair.

Even without knowing how to interpret all the nuances of this dream, you can probably detect Colleen's worries about her appearance and loss of attractiveness to her husband. When we discussed this in class, the other students pointed out that, if she wanted to have this baby, Colleen must accept her increased weight and bodily changes. Experienced mothers also attested to the ease in regaining one's figure, particularly for a woman who was in such excellent condition when she conceived.

Another first-timer pointed out, "I see this as a time to

indulge myself once in awhile. I never used to eat ice cream; now I treat myself occasionally, figuring I'll lose the extra pound or so after the baby comes." One of the husbands commented, "I certainly don't expect my wife to look like a fashion model for the next nine months. Her belly getting bigger just reassures us that the baby is growing and it makes me proud. I just love her all the more."

THE POSITIVE STATEMENT AND DAYDREAM

As a way to learn to accept the changes brought about by pregnancy, we suggested that Colleen take one of her negative body image thoughts and create a positive daydream with it. She closed her eyes, took several long, deliberate breaths, exhaled slowly each time, and then reversed her feelings. "I hate the way my waistline is getting thicker" became "My baby is growing and making my body more beautiful."

Colleen now had the basis for an affirmation that could help her prevent any future negative thoughts about her figure. Using this positive statement as the "plot" of her daydream, she let herself imagine the best possible way for her husband Carl to aid her in developing a better body image. Then she opened her eyes and, imagining that someone was describing the scene to her, wrote the following:

> Looking in the mirror at yourself, you see the new curve of your belly and the way your waist is getting wider. You smile and think, "Our baby is growing inside." Then your husband Carl comes in and stands behind you. He gently touches your swollen belly and kisses the nape of your neck. He whispers, "You're more beautiful than ever." You feel the baby kick, and you press Carl's hand onto your stomach. "It's moving!" you tell him. "Can you feel it kick?" Carl kneels down and puts his ear against your belly. "I can hear the heartbeat!" he says excitedly. He

stands up and takes you in his arms and kisses you, telling you again how beautiful you are and how much he loves you and the baby.

INTEGRATING THE CREATIVE DAYDREAM

In order to impress this beautiful daydream on her deeper consciousness, Colleen was instructed in a simple relaxation technique that summoned up the powers of her inner consciousness. Deep relaxation is essential in order to become aware of the imaginative thoughts our right brains constantly generate.

With our muscles at ease, many beneficial physical effects occur, such as lowered blood pressure and heart rate. Right brain images and pictures also provide us with powerful, creative ideas and effective solutions for conflicts or problems.

After Colleen became deeply relaxed, another student read her the daydream she had composed. Carl repeated it to her when she got home. The next week Colleen told us: "All this caused some kind of breakthrough in our relationship. Now, I feel Carl is really with me 100 percent. All of a sudden, just by sharing this problem with me, he seems to understand why I've been worried, and he's really letting me know how much he wants this baby."

To integrate your own positive affirmations and daydreams, you may want to have your partner read the daydream aloud after you're relaxed. Or you might find it helpful to speak the words into a tape recorder and play them back to yourself during a peaceful moment.

Relaxation Techniques

Whatever method you use, the most important part of the procedure is to learn to relax deeply. Although there are many excellent audio cassettes for relaxation available, I recommend that you use my instructions to make your own. My relaxation methods are designed specifically for pregnancy, and will do more than help you relax. They will also teach you to use the various sets of muscles in your body that play an important part in labor and delivery. These same relaxation methods are recommended by the eminent British childbirth educator Dr. Sheila Kitzinger and are taught to instructors certified by the International Childbirth Educators Association (ICEA). While somewhat different from Lamaze methods, they do not conflict in any way. My adapted relaxation techniques result from several years' experience with expectant parents.

You may want your partner to read the following instructions onto your tape, so that you can hear his voice when he's not with you. At times when you study together, he will be able to direct you personally. Most women find that they relax more easily when a voice other than their own provides the instructions. Should this be inconvenient, however, you can read onto the tape yourself and play it back at another time.

The two simple relaxation techniques I use are called "Progressive Relaxation" and "Autogenic Training." They will help you relieve any stress you may encounter.

Although they seem alike at first glance, these two techniques actually have slightly different effects on the depth of relaxation most pregnant women experience when employing them. Progressive Relaxation, with its emphasis on control of each set of muscles in your body, is usually not sleep-inducing. Autogenic Training, on the other hand, frequently relaxes you so completely that you nod off, sometimes before finishing the exercises.

By the way, these relaxation methods can be used effectively by anyone, female or male, pregnant or not. Once you have learned the process, you may want to share it with your partner. He can also benefit from these simple procedures to relieve tension.

PROGRESSIVE RELAXATION

With this technique you deliberately tighten, contract, and then release every set of muscles in your body, one at a time. Our muscles tighten when under stress; Progressive Relaxation effectively interrupts the tense-mind, tense-muscle cycle. The technique derives its name from the orderly system for progressively easing stress from head to toe. When working with pregnant women, I have found this method most helpful for integrating positive thoughts and affirmations into the deeper consciousness. By concentrating on the simple exercises for each muscle set, your left brain becomes calm, allowing your right hemisphere to absorb the images it will receive from your taped creative daydream.

Prepare for Progressive Relaxation by choosing a warm, private room—perhaps bedroom, livingroom, or dining area. Since cool or cold air may prevent muscle relaxation, however, it is best to choose a comfortably heated and relatively draft-free place. Avoid distractions; be sure the telephone is disconnected and there are as few outside noises as possible.

Collect several pillows and lie down on a bed, sofa, or the floor, if it's carpeted or covered with a rug. Arrange the cushions around and under your body, until the environment simulates a cozy, relaxing nest. Some pregnant women like one or two small toss pillows under their knees. If you are more at ease on your side, by all means get in that position.

Now you are ready to play the tape carrying the instructions below:

Take three long, deep, cleansing breaths. Inhale through your nose and exhale very slowly through your mouth. With each breath, let go of any distracting thoughts. There's nothing to do now, no place to go, nothing that has to be done until later. Just relax . . . relax . . . relax.

Now bring your attention to your face. Tighten all your facial muscles, screw up your face, squint your eyes tightly shut. As you do this, take a breath and hold it for the count of three: one . . . two . . . three. Now let the breath out and relax your face. Notice the difference. Close your eyes and enjoy the relaxed feeling in your whole face.

With your eyes still closed, think about your neck and shoulders. Take a breath and tighten the muscles in your neck and shoulders. Hold the tightness and your breath for the count of three. One . . . two . . . three. Now, exhale and let the tightness in your neck and shoulders relax. Notice the difference.

Next, concentrate on your buttocks and lower back. Take a breath and tighten your buttocks. Arch your back and feel the tightness. Hold this tension for the count of three. One . . . two . . . three. Let the breath out normally, allowing your buttocks and lower back to relax. Notice the difference. Check your face and neck and shoulders. If they are tightening up again, take another quick breath, tense them, hold the tension for three counts, and then release. Now your body is becoming more and more relaxed.

Think about your abdomen. Inhaling, tighten your stomach muscles and hold for the count of three. One . . . two . . . three. Release the breath and the tightness. Place one hand on your belly and tighten these muscles again as you take a breath. Hold for the count of three. Exhale and relax your abdomen. Let your hand feel the difference.

Move your attention to your thighs. Inhaling, tighten your thigh muscles. Hold for three counts. One . . . two . . . three. Release breath and tension. Notice your relaxed thighs.

Concentrate on your calf muscles. Take a breath and tighten these muscles. Hold for three counts. One . . . two . . . three. Let the breath and the tightness out. Now your calf muscles are relaxed.

Take a breath and tighten your feet and ankles by flexing

both feet with the toes pointing back toward your head. You may feel your whole leg tighten. Hold the tension for three. One . . . two . . . three. Now let your breath out and allow your legs and feet to relax.

Make fists with both hands. Inhale and tighten each arm from shoulders to fingertips. Make both arms very rigid. Feel your biceps tightening. Hold the breath as you count to three. One . . . two . . . three. Now release and let your arms flop to your sides. Breathe normally and stretch your fingers until they're totally relaxed.

With your eyes still closed, imagine each set of muscles from your head to your toes. If any sets of muscles are at all tense, release them now. Stretch your toes to be sure they're also relaxed.

Now that you feel totally at ease, listen to your new daydream. The most effective way to do this is to hear it being read aloud to you. Ideally, your partner should repeat it in a soft, gentle voice. If that is inconvenient, a tape of either him or you will be equally effective.

Some pregnant women find that they are able to open their eyes and simply read the daydream to themselves, silently. However, the most important variable remains deep relaxation. If opening your eyes and reading it brings you back to an overly alert state, listen to a tape or to your partner.

Other women have told me that all they needed to do was to become relaxed and silently review the daydream from memory. This easy absorption may be due to the somewhat altered state of consciousness often encountered during pregnancy. This mood is completely natural, a kind of heightened awareness of right-brain images, making you more open to suggestions than when you were not pregnant.

Whatever fashion you choose to integrate your positive, affirmative daydream, *be sure to follow these directions prior to getting up:*

Imagine the way the room looked before you began your relaxation practice. Picture the lighting, the furniture, and the area where you're resting. Allow your body to feel the surface beneath you. This will help you avoid a sense of shock upon returning to "reality."

Silently repeat to yourself, "I am relaxed and refreshed. When I get up, I will feel alert and rested." This exercise eliminates the lingering effects of drowsiness when you arise. Also, giving yourself this suggestion while deeply relaxed encourages your brain to send appropriate signals to your body; you soon will feel clear-headed and revitalized.

Yawn and stretch. Slowly open your eyes and blink them a few times.

Sit up. Shake your hands as if they were limp dishrags. Stretch and yawn again.

If you were resting on the floor, do this step next. (If you were on a bed or couch, skip to the next paragraph.) Place your hands on the floor and lean over into a squatting position. Push your weight back onto your heels as you slowly roll your body up into a standing position. Stretch and yawn once more. Shake your hands and fingers out again to bring blood circulation away from your head. This will prevent you from feeling dizzy or disoriented.

If you were resting on a bed or couch, swing your legs around so they touch the floor. Stand up slowly and then shake out your hands and fingers again. Stretch and yawn once more. Coming back to your waking world in this gradual, gentle manner will get your blood circulating away from your head, avoiding dizziness and preparing you to engage in normal activities.

Autogenic Training

The technique of Autogenic Training is especially helpful to people who suffer from insomnia. Many pregnant women complain that they have difficulty going back to sleep after waking from a nightmare, bathroom trip, or fetal movements. If insomnia bothers you, Autogenic Training can be a valuable tool.

Autogenic Training techniques, like those of Progressive Relaxation, focus on each body part: face, neck, shoulders, lower back, and arms. However, the effects differ markedly. In Progressive Relaxation, your attention was brought to each set of muscles in the various areas of the body: the muscles around your eyes, in your neck and shoulders, etc. You also were instructed to tighten and then release those muscles.

In Autogenic Training you learn to *begin* by focusing on the body parts that you imagine are *already* relaxed, heavy, and warm. This technique usually results in such deep relaxation that many pregnant women fall asleep—often before the end of the instructions! Evidently the repeated suggestions of heaviness and warmth are so effective that the waking mind simply "checks out."

Try Autogenic Training just before going to bed, when the stresses of the day often linger and keep us awake. The technique is also beneficial when you feel tense or anxious.

Some of my students prefer Autogenic Training when they're integrating positive daydreams and affirmations. If you can stay awake, you may want to try it with your own daydreams. To do this, wait until the end of the exercises. Then review your creative daydream in one of the ways described above for Progressive Relaxation.

To practice Autogenic Training, prepare yourself just as you did for Progressive Relaxation. When you're comfortable, listen to these procedures:

Take three long, deep, cleansing breaths by inhaling through your nose and exhaling *very slowly* through your mouth. With each breath, let go of any distracting thoughts. There's nothing to do now, no place to go, nothing that has to be done until later. Just relax . . . relax . . . relax.

Allow your eyelids to close. Silently repeat to yourself, "My eyelids feel heavy and warm. My eyelids feel heavy and warm." Imagine that all you can see is inky blackness. If you cannot imagine blackness, picture a white screen instead. Imagine that you are pouring black India ink onto the white screen so that it gradually becomes totally black.

Let the warmth and heaviness from your eyes spread down onto all of your face. Let it spread over your nose, cheeks, mouth, and jaw. Tell yourself, "My entire face feels heavy and warm. My face feels heavy and warm." Don't *try* to make anything feel heavy and warm, just notice what happens as you say these words to yourself.

Now let the relaxation spread down into your throat, your neck, and your shoulders. Repeat to yourself, "My neck and shoulders are heavy and warm. My neck and shoulders are heavy and warm."

Breathe deeply through your nose and slowly out of your mouth as you count to eight. With each count, the warmth and heaviness spreads into your chest and upper back. One . . . two . . . three . . . heavier and warmer . . . four . . . five . . . six . . . more and more relaxed . . . seven . . . eight. Now you're deeply relaxed. In a moment you'll open your eyes and close them again.

At the count of three, you'll open your eyes to test their heaviness. One . . . two . . . three. Now, open your eyes and notice how heavy they feel. You want to close them. Now close your eyes and notice how heavy and warm your eyelids feel. That relaxation has spread down your face, your neck, your shoulders, and into your chest and upper back.

Tell yourself, "Both of my arms feel heavy and warm. Both my arms feel heavy and warm." Let the warmth and heaviness spread into your hands. Let it extend through your fingertips. Now, both of your arms and hands feel heavy and warm.

The relaxation spreads into your abdomen. Repeat to

yourself, "My stomach feels heavy and warm. My stomach feels heavy and warm. All the organs in my abdomen feel heavy and warm. All the organs in my abdomen feel heavy and warm." Now tell yourself, "My lower back feels heavy and warm. My lower back feels heavy and warm." Now your lower back is deeply relaxed. Repeat to yourself, "My thighs are heavy and warm. Both my thighs are heavy and warm." Let the relaxation spread over your knees and into your calves. Tell yourself, "The calves of my legs feel heavy and warm. The calves of my legs feel heavy and warm." The heaviness and warmth are spreading into your ankles and feet. Repeat to yourself, "My feet and toes are heavy and warm. My feet and toes are heavy and warm." Now the relaxation has spread from your eyes all the way down to your toes. Let all the tension trickle out of your toes. Mentally check your entire body. If your scalp feels tight, tell yourself it feels heavy and warm. If any part of your body feels tight, stop at that place and tell yourself that it feels heavy and warm. Heavy and warm.

If you wish to impress any positive thought or daydream on your deeper consciousness, now is the time to repeat those thoughts or words.

If you want to go to sleep, this is the time to tell yourself, "I am drifting off into a deep, relaxing, refreshing sleep. I will remember my dreams when I wake up. When I wake up, I'll remember my dreams. I am drifting off into a deep, relaxing, refreshing sleep. When I wake up, I'll remember my dreams."

If you do not wish to fall asleep, skip the previous paragraph and follow the same instructions at the end of the Progressive Relaxation method. Be sure to come back into "reality" very slowly, and as you stand up, shake out your hands and fingers to bring blood circulation away from your head.

Results of Step 1

Most of the pregnant women who have studied my five-step program are amazed at the changes that occur at this first, simple stage. Miranda, a 29-year-old TV production assistant in her second trimester, told me, "The day after I started keeping my diary, I remembered two nightmares. It was uncanny that they both seemed to be about the very same negative thoughts I'd written down before falling asleep! I'd been worrying about a new script girl who has her eye on my job." These are Miranda's dream records:

> *Dream #1:* I'm on a ship that's going down. Everyone is rushing for the lifeboats and there aren't enough. I manage to squeeze into one and as it's lowered, Cindy (the new woman on our show) jumps in. She lands right on top of me and starts pushing me out. The boat is rocking in high waves and I go overboard. I'm yelling at the others to make her stop. I shout, "Can't you see I'm pregnant?" but they pay no attention. Then I woke up with my heart pounding.

> *Dream #2:* I'm shopping at Macy's, standing in line at the cashier's with a lot of bundles. Layette things. A woman I don't know pushes in at the front of the line and the rest of us start complaining. One woman says, "She isn't even in the right department. She's not even buying baby things." I feel annoyed but don't say anything.

Although Miranda had not yet learned how to interpret all the symbols of these dreams, she immediately realized they reflected her concern about being replaced when she went on maternity leave. "The first thing I noticed," she commented, "was that the 'villain' in both my dreams was *pushing* me out of the way. That's just the way I feel about Cindy at work. And both dreams show me this is all somehow connected to my pregnancy."

Even though she didn't believe it would actually help, Miranda reversed her negative thought ("I'm worried I may lose my job to Cindy when I go on maternity leave") to a positive one ("I can handle my career and being a mother"). Next, she pictured herself successfully engaged in both pursuits. She then wrote the following creative daydream for her partner to read to her after she became deeply relaxed:

> You are at home with our new baby, who is sleeping peacefully. You call the office and Cindy answers. She tells you about what's been happening while you've been away, and then your boss gets on. He congratulates you and says, "Don't worry about your job, Miranda. We really need you here. As soon as you can, maybe you'd like to come in part-time. Or, you can take some work home with you."

After integrating this affirmative daydream, Miranda approached her employer about job guarantees. As it turned out, that particular TV network provided female staff with a three-month maternity leave and assurance that their jobs would be held for at least as long.

By confronting her fears and taking action, Miranda found a quick resolution. "I was getting tied up in knots over nothing," she said. "If my dreams hadn't warned me, I could have gone for months worrying about something that never would have happened. Also, the entire incident made me more aware of employees' rights, so now I'm attending all the network's human resources committee meetings. The parents among us are working to set up a daycare center for infants too young for nursery school."

Jaimie, a 30-year-old homemaker with 2-year-old twins, was another of my students who got immediate relief after beginning to record her dreams and negative thoughts. In her fourth month of the current pregnancy, she had the following nightmare:

> I'm in a restaurant having lunch with the twins and my mother. We're having trouble keeping the boys quiet because some people across the way have brought a puppy into the restaurant. The boys are so excited they won't sit

still, and they keep teasing the pup with bits of food. It yips and jumps around. The couple with the dog say to us, "It's inconsiderate to bring small children into a restaurant." Mom gets mad and tells them, "You're no one to talk! Animals aren't allowed in here!" Then Bob (my husband) comes in and shouts, "This place is on fire! Hurry and get out!" The smoke is pouring in and we're coughing. Bob and Mom and I try to get the twins out of their high chairs when that puppy runs over. His leash gets tangled up around the chair legs. He starts biting the boys and barking. I manage to get one of the boys loose and start for the door. Someone pushes me down and then I woke up, so upset I had to go look in on the boys to be sure they were okay.

When Jaimie recorded this dream, she did not know that small animals usually symbolize the unborn child in pregnant women's dreams. Jaimie voiced her concern: "I think it's about my worry that I'm never going to be able to manage another baby so soon. Mom will come and help out for the first month, but even so, I'm already feeling overwhelmed."

Then Leah, another mother of a 2-year-old, asked, "Are you worried that the new baby will upset your boys the way the puppy did in your dreams? I know I am. I'm afraid my little boy won't understand when I tell him I still love him. He'll see me nursing and just be hurt and jealous." This discussion led Jaimie to realize that, like most women with other children, she, too, was anxious about the effect the new baby would have on its siblings.

Both Jaimie and Leah put their heads together and came up with a creative daydream to help them overcome their shared anxiety:

You're about to nurse the new baby. First, you get your older boy(s) onto the bed with you, one on each side, with bottled juice. Then you begin nursing, all the while cuddling with your older boy(s). He (they) stroke the baby as you guide the little hands, teaching gentleness. You sing a lullaby and the older one(s) join in. All the children fall asleep and your husband comes in, picks up the baby and burps him, and you sigh with happiness.

When they read this daydream aloud in class, Leah and Jaimie got a few laughs. "Don't you wish it could really be that idyllic!" someone jeered. Nevertheless, both worried mothers were able to ease their anxiety and continued to make plans for staving off any possible sibling rivalry. In a few weeks Jaimie commented, "Just getting this worry out in the open and trying to think of ways I can cope has helped a lot. Somehow, I know we can manage and I feel more confident about mothering three little ones."

Practicing Step 1

The first step in this program simply requires you to write down your dreams immediately upon awakening. Make sure your partner and any other family members permit you a few moments of uninterrupted privacy each morning. You will also need to purchase some sort of notebook or diary to be used as your dream diary.

Every night before going to bed, enter the date at the top of a page and briefly record any negative thoughts you have had that day. Then choose one of these thoughts and reverse it into a positive statement. After writing down your dreams the following day, you will create a fantasy, using the positive statement from the previous night as a "plot." Finally, practice one of the two relaxation techniques and then either listen to a tape recording or repeat your positive daydream to yourself. This will integrate the fantasy into your deeper consciousness.

Having learned how to keep your dream diary and to reverse your negative thoughts into affirmative, creative visions, you are ready to study some of the even more fascinating aspects of your dreams, their symbols and interpretations.

CHAPTER 4

❖

Step 2: Interpreting Your Dream Symbols and Diagramming Your Dreams

Zelda, a 30-year-old Boston travel agent in her fifth month, wrote the following:

> The article about your study of pregnant women's dreams mentioned that we often dream about former boyfriends and lovers. Also, that small animals mean the dream is about the baby. Last night I dreamed this: I was in a tropical jungle, on a kind of safari with the guy I went steady with in high school. I wasn't pregnant in the dream. The trees and the ground were just teeming with all kinds of little animals—cute little monkeys hanging by their tails and jabbering at us, colorful birds chirping and singing, lizards and snakes sliding by, not bothering us, making me laugh and feel happy. Lots of huge, sweet-smelling blossoms everywhere. I kept tripping over leafy vines. We made camp and this boyfriend killed a rabbit and began to skin it for our dinner. I felt nauseous and woke up feeling like really throwing up. My questions

are: if small animals are symbols of my baby, does the
skinned rabbit mean something will happen to my baby,
or that I'll have to have a C-section? And, I'm dreaming
a lot about this old lover, even though we quarreled and
I haven't seen him for years. Does this mean that, some-
where deep inside, I really love him and not my husband?
I love this guy in my dreams, but in real life my husband
comes first.

This expectant mother needn't have worried about any
harm coming to her unborn child. Even though the slaugh-
tered rabbit appears foreboding, this incident in Zelda's
otherwise pleasant dream only represented her fear that
something might go wrong. Actually, she wrote me later
that she gave birth to a healthy, eight-pound, six-ounce
baby boy. Her uncomplicated labor had lasted merely six
hours.

The other small animals in Zelda's dream were portrayed
as lively, happy creatures, probably indicative of the way
Zelda usually imagined her unborn child. Despite the recent
scientific findings of dream researchers, many people cling to
misconceptions about dream symbols.

Dream Symbols

Webster's Seventh New Collegiate Dictionary defines a
symbol as "something that stands for or suggests something
else by reason of relationship, association, convention, or
accidental resemblance, *esp:* a visible sign of something in-
visible." A *dream symbol* is an image or a picture in a dream,
which usually stands for something else in the dreamer's
waking life.

Sometimes dreams featuring characters or settings from
the pregnant woman's past appear to be attempts to review
previously successful strategies for the resolution of problems. Thus, Zelda's frequent dreams about her former boy-

friend may have reminded her that the two of them enjoyed some activities that were missing in her current relationship. Acting on this dream suggestion, Zelda then encouraged her husband to try different sorts of recreation. "He was missing not being able to go out dancing and partying all night," she wrote. "So now we're doing healthier things together like taking long walks and going to museums. And it's really more fun, at least for now."

THE ORIGIN OF DREAM SYMBOLS

According to the theory proposed by Dr. John Antrobus, many of our dream experiences originate in the same portion of the brain that functions when we're awake. These are called the "cognitive" aspects of dreams, plots or stories leaving us with the uncanny feeling of actually participating in the episode. Upon awakening, it is the now more alert part of the mind's task to translate these images into understandable language. The late British psychologist Christopher Evans speculated that our brains constantly rewrite existing computer-like "programs" to help explain the day's experiences.

Although dream symbols are unique to each individual, certain groups of people seem to have similar dreams and repeatedly tell researchers of identical or very similar symbolic meanings. This phenomenon especially holds true for some women who share the same stage of physical development.

For instance, Dr. Robert Van de Castle found remarkably similar themes in the menstrual-cycle dreams of females of a like age, educational background, and career level. Dr. Patricia Garfield's most recent book, *Women's Bodies, Women's Dreams,* emphasizes the dream similarities of women as they go through various stages of physical and mental maturation, from childhood and puberty to the post-menopausal years.

SPECIAL QUALITIES OF PREGNANCY DREAM SYMBOLS

The dreams of pregnancy also have many parallels, regardless of the backgrounds and past experiences of the individual dreamers. When I noticed the repetition of certain symbols in the dream journals of my volunteers, I interviewed them to determine their personal associations. For instance, a majority of the pregnant women surveyed mentioned dreams of water in some form—from the powerful ocean to leaking water heaters, overflowing toilets, and plain old baths. Still, each one mentioned that water brought to mind something about pregnancy or childbirth.

These same associations rarely, if ever, occur to *nonexpectant* people. For example, to expectant parents, dreams of taking a trip or going on a journey usually symbolize the pregnancy and its progress through time toward the delivery. However, nonexpectant people often associate trips and journeys with diverse events in their waking lives, such as changing jobs or the transitions from one relationship to another (marriage to divorce).

EXCEPTIONS TO PREGNANCY DREAM SYMBOLS

A word of caution: although expectant parents frequently derive similar meanings from dream symbols, *this may not always be the case.* For instance, dream researchers tell us that the cuddly kittens, puppies, or bunnies imagined during early pregnancy usually stand for the fetus. Yet Agnes, one of the pregnant women I interviewed, interpreted a stampede by hundreds of bunnies as her fear of sex. She told me she associated rabbits with sex and worried that having intercourse might somehow hurt the baby.

I reassured Agnes that she need not deny herself and her husband the pleasures of intercourse during pregnancy and gave her some literature on the topic. If I had assumed her dream merely meant that she was perhaps feeling overwhelmed by her pregnancy—a reasonable interpretation if we believe that bunnies symbolize the fetus—then she might never have told me about the secret fear that was already causing needless misunderstanding between her and her puzzled mate.

Therefore, when interpreting dream symbols, always examine the individual's associations with each image or symbol. Bear in mind that pregnant women of the same general age group often have similar bodily and hormonal changes, frequently share concerns about issues and problems, and usually attach like meanings to their dream symbols. To better understand your own dreams, you may want to jot down your own associations as you read the following list.

Common Symbols in Pregnancy Dreams

Each of the general categories or meanings listed below is followed by a group of its most common dream symbols.

Your baby or fetus, especially in early pregnancy. *Plants* (flowers, shrubs, bushes, gardens); *small animals* (birds, kittens, puppies, gophers, worms, mice, fish, lizards); *human babies, a child, children, or you, yourself as a child.*

Your baby or fetus, especially in late pregnancy. *Large plants* (vines, trees, parks, vineyards, orchards, jungles, extravagant botanical scenes) indicate the growing life within; *large animals* (dogs, wolves, tigers, lions, dinosaurs) are more frequent in the dreams of pregnant women having other children, with the animals often attacking the older children.

You. *You as an infant or child,* especially in early pregnancy dreams, when you may not be able to visualize yourself caring for a tiny infant; sometimes *your mother,* with whom you may identify quite strongly; *yourself in the recent past,* probably indicates either ambivalence about your pregnancy and a wish to return to other times, or an attempt to review the way you handled a previous problem; *vehicles* (automobiles, boats, planes, ships, bikes, trains, trucks, wagons) suggest your body as it moves through pregnancy.

Transition to motherhood. *Clothing, shopping for larger clothes; catastrophes* (deaths, funerals, other disasters) all indicate an awareness that your life-style is changing dramatically; *intruders* (including burglars, muggers, threatening strangers, and monsters) suggest that you see something about your pregnancy as dangerous or life-threatening.

Your womb. *Architectural references* (including rooms, houses, larger buildings, skyscrapers) may become larger and more complicated as your waistline expands; much emphasis on *basements,* sometimes filled with *tunnels* and *mazes,* suggests the birth canal; *underground dwellings, caves, and caverns* also indicate the uterus.

Your pregnancy. *Any growing things,* including gardens and jungles, may also portray the baby; *journeys, hikes, exercise, climbing, swimming, running, or other movements and actions* suggest progress toward a goal (delivery and birth).

Labor and delivery. *Water* portrays the amniotic fluid in which the fetus is suspended or the "waters breaking" at the onset of labor; in early pregnancy, water symbols may include *puddles, bathtubs, or overflowing toilets;* later, water is depicted as *swimming pools, lakes, rain, storms, and oceans,* with the wavelike activity representing the ebb and flow of labor contractions; *scenes of death and environmental disasters* such as earthquakes, fires, and storms, as well as *robbers, threatening strangers, or rapists,* may reflect a fear of harm to the baby or a complicated delivery; if the intruders wield sharp instruments or knives, this may mean you fear a C-section or some other medical intervention; *hospitals, doctors, and nurses* all indicate the delivery; *actual delivery scenes,* if frightening, usually reflect needless anxiety; dreams of an abnormally *easy deliv-*

ery, where the baby simply "pops out" with little or no effort on your part, may suggest an unwillingness to accept the possibility that the delivery will bring pain or discomfort; *barriers* (including fences, walls, mazes, and other obstructions) could indicate that you anticipate labor as a tremendous hurdle.

Nurturing, breast-feeding, caring for the newborn. *Eating* (including food, cooking, shopping for food, visiting restaurants).

Fear of loss of your mate. *Clothing* too small or unbecoming; dreams of *a rival* or scenes of your partner having an affair or leaving with *another woman* may mean that you perceive yourself as unattractive.

Relatives. *Members of your family* indicate your desire for harmony and a resolution of any familial conflicts; *your mother*—or *an authoritative figure* such as a teacher or older friend representing your mother—may suggest the way you actually feel about her or about some conflict in your current relationship; she may represent you yourself as a mother, or a fear you may make the same mistakes in parenting as your mother did with you; dreams of *your partner* (husband, mate, the expectant father) usually reflect your true feelings about him; sometimes your *father* may symbolize your partner; or your father may be in your dreams to suggest that you need to resolve some old conflict with him; a *nurse* sometimes depicts a relative, or perhaps yourself as a caregiver.

Emotions. *Feelings* in dreams are usually not symbolic but instead are clues to the way you perceive a situation in your waking life; *sexual feelings* sometimes indicate a reliving of the conception or a desire for more intimacy with your partner; *painful or unpleasant sexual scenes* suggest an ambivalence about your pregnancy, as if your body has been invaded by something unpleasant or painful.

Working expectant mothers. *Your boss, colleagues, co-workers, or office* usually represent some concern about balancing your job or career and motherhood; a *physician or other authoritative figure* may symbolize your employer—or perhaps your father or husband—depending upon how you feel about these people in your waking life.

Having read this list of typical symbols and themes in pregnant women's dreams, you may already have some good ideas about the meaning of your own dreams. Please remember one important fact: the first meaning that occurs to you is probably the correct one. Trust your spontaneous thoughts and go with your own translation, even if the objects, emotions, or characters you associate with any part of your dream do not match those given in the list above. Ask yourself, "What does this remind me of in my waking life?"

INTERPRETING DREAM SYMBOLS

In every dream, your deeper consciousness, your dreaming self, sends you symbolic messages. This is the reason for writing down even a fragment of a dream, if that's all you recall.

As you read the following dream, look for small animals representing the fetus and for other pregnancy birth symbols. Also look for architectural references indicating the woman's body or womb. Notice the dreamer's relatives and try to guess how she feels about them. It will also be helpful for you to know that Hazel, the 30-year-old homemaker who reported this dream in her fourth month, had a history of miscarriages before this pregnancy.

> My husband and I are walking under an overpass. There are people and chickens everywhere. It's almost as if it were a park. I see my parents sitting on the hood of a car. My father has a can of soda pop in his hand and is laying

his head on my mother's shoulder. She has her arm around his back. They're relaxed and cuddling together. (My parents haven't cuddled for at least eight years, maybe more! Right now, they're getting a divorce.) Then a cat runs ahead of us and chases a chicken but never catches up to it. We come to a green, grassy, sloping hilly sort of place where we see a giant chicken coop. It is built on an "A" type of design or pyramid. The inside is nice too. The whole building is constructed of canvas and wood. The "head" chicken sends out an alarm or call to a conference of some sort. All the chickens everywhere start going to the hen house. It is amazing! She keeps calling that call and they keep coming!

This dream contains many symbols referring to the fetus and childbirth. For example, the underpass is a tunnel-like structure, possibly symbolizing the birth canal. Chickens and the cat may be fetal depictions. The park and the grassy, sloping hills are symbols of growing things. The "head" chicken probably is a "mother hen," symbolizing maternity. The architectural symbol of the chicken coop may represent Hazel's expanding uterus.

Notice Hazel's comments about her parents. It's clear that she wished they were happy together, so that her baby would arrive in a closely knit, harmonious family. Hazel also thought this dream had a special meaning, with the mother hen calling all the chicks to roost. She said, "I'm healthy now and ready for all those babies I wasn't able to carry before." In actuality, Hazel became pregnant again quite soon after this first child was born.

Two months later, during her sixth month, Hazel reported the following dream:

We (a guy I went to elementary school with) were going on a date. We walked up and down many outdoor stairways, going past many different restaurants. One was all Victorian. Even the wallpaper was authentic. Another was very elegant with sterling silver and lead crystal place settings. When we got to our restaurant it looked like a run-down villa in Mexico. It was on a lot with dirt, no grass, and dried up trees and plants. It was adobe. We went inside and it was very nice (to my surprise and relief). We were eating when my husband came walking by and informed me he was checking out the place to rent it. I knew I should be doing that, too, and got up to look around. Found a room that had a door hung sideways on a wall. There was a fireplace inside. When you didn't want a fire, you dropped the door. I called, "Honey, it has a fireplace!" and woke up.

Notice how the architectural references continue to be important symbols in Hazel's dreams. The pyramid-shaped hen house of her earlier dream appears simple compared to the elaborate restaurants she and her old boyfriend encounter; since this dream occurred two months after the henhouse dream, Hazel's body has no doubt changed: her uterus has become larger and its contents (the fetus and the nurturing fluids surrounding it) more complex.

The building Hazel and her dream companion finally enter is the least attractive of all, on the outside. She thought this symbolized her self-concept at this stage of her pregnancy. Hazel and her husband had just begun attending Lamaze classes and she confided, "I actually wished I looked *more* pregnant, that my belly was bigger, so I would be more like the other women in the class. But I'm just naturally skinny, so I don't show much yet."

Hazel said that her former boyfriends appeared in most of her dreams. Unlike Zelda, she didn't worry about this. "I know my marriage is the best ever," she explained, "and these old lovers just come around so I can check them out and see once more how terrific my husband is, in comparison!"

By examining the action and plot of her dream, Hazel saw that even though she perceived herself as "not lush enough, sorta dried up, like the adobe restaurant," her husband held a different opinion. He was eagerly planning for the new baby, depicted in the dream as his house-hunting effort.

Hazel commented, "We both know our baby is in there, warm and cozy, just like the fireplace behind the door."

To give you an idea of the marvelous variety of dream symbols, here are some excerpts from other pregnant women's dreams:

Anjelika, 32-year-old florist, in her fourth month: All the pansies in a bouquet I was preparing became babies' faces.

Mattie, 30-year-old art gallery director, in her ninth month: We lived in a house perched dangerously high on a cliff, overlooking the ocean. There was a raging storm. We hid in the basement and I was surprised at all the rooms down there. The waves flooded the house.

Tanya, 26-year-old actress in her sixth month: Dreamt I was taking a bubble bath . . . the tub lifted up, flew right out the window, landed on a lake. As it was sinking, I noticed there were all kinds of live animals in the tub: little ducks, chicks, some goldfish, and a spotted puppy.

Josephine, 28-year-old homemaker, in her eighth month: My stepdaughter came running in, crying. She said my collie dog was "making doo doo" all over her dolls. (Actually, that dog died years ago.)

Anjelika's dream of the flowers with babies' faces was a lovely reflection of the growing life she carried within and typical of an early pregnancy dream. The cliff house, on the other hand, indicated different perceptions of pregnancy as Mattie neared her due date. She commented, "I feel as if I'm on the brink of something dangerous—the delivery, I guess." Notice too, the ocean, the raging storm, the flooding waves, all indications of impending labor. Mattie's basement, symbolizing her womb, contained many rooms, just as her uterus was now brimming with the fully formed fetus.

Tanya's dream of the flying bathtub is also filled with delivery symbols (the lake and the sinking tub suggest her anxiety about not being able to get through the labor) and fetal symbols (little ducks, chicks, goldfish, the puppy). Typical of both late pregnancy and multiparous dreams, Josephine sees her unborn child (the large collie) as a possible threat to her stepdaughter's feelings of security. Having studied a variety of symbols, you are ready to discover how this knowledge can be used to interpret your dreams. My diagramming technique highlights these dream symbols for easy analysis.

Diagramming Your Dreams

Please don't be put off by the technical sound of the word "diagramming." This method is so easy that you'll be amazed at the way the elements of any dream will begin to make sense. Simply circle all the dream symbols you can find and underline all the action words (verbs).

To practice this method, let's look at two dreams that Janet and her husband Eric had on the same night. It will help us to know that this couple just started attending their Lamaze classes. Here is Eric's dream:

> My wife Janet and I were in a rowboat on a quiet lake. It was a peaceful, sunny day. We were taking turns with the oars when suddenly the sky darkened and it began to rain very hard. Janet began clutching her belly and yelling that the baby was coming. I tried not to panic but we were a long way from shore. She was screaming for me to help her and I was trying to row us back. The storm got worse, with lightning and thunder. Huge waves nearly capsized us. I woke up in a sweat. The dream was so real I had to check to see if Janet was okay. She's in her sixth month and everything is fine, but that dream really shook me up!

This is Janet's dream:

> In this dream I am floating on my back in a swimming pool on a large cruise ship. The water is warm and I feel very happy because the water sort of buoys me up. My stom-

ach is looming over me because I am very pregnant. I am so big, I can't see my toes. But I feel safe because everything is very calm. Then I notice all the other swimmers are also pregnant. I notice the lifeguard and realize it is Eric. Then alarm bells and sirens start up, making a horrible, deafening noise. At first I think it is a drill but the sky gets black, icy raindrops hit my skin, and the ship begins to roll. Big waves rise up in the pool. Some of the women start screaming and trying to get out. But I can't move! I try to turn over but my stomach is too heavy. I try to kick but can't feel anything. I get a mouthful of water and start to choke. Eric throws in a ring but I can't reach it. I realize he is too busy with everyone screaming and milling around and that he can't help me. (At this point I woke up, feeling terrified.)

From what you've just read about dream symbols, you will have guessed that these landlubbers envisioned boats, ships, lakes, a swimming pool, and a storm at sea because these aquatic images symbolized the pregnancy, impending labor, and delivery.

Now you'll discover how much more you can learn from your dreams by simply diagramming them. First, circle all the symbols. These should include the setting, objects, and characters. Next, underline all the action words or the main verbs. This allows you a clear look at both the content and the action of the dream, as well as the ways these elements interact.

When Eric diagrammed his dream, it looked like this:

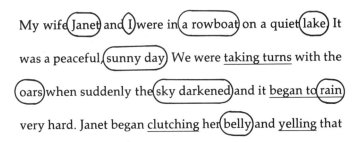

My wife (Janet) and (I) were in (a rowboat) on a quiet (lake) It was a peaceful (sunny day) We were taking turns with the (oars) when suddenly the (sky darkened) and it began to (rain) very hard. Janet began clutching her (belly) and yelling that the (baby) was coming. I <u>tried not to panic</u> but we were a

long way from (shore.) She was <u>screaming</u> for me <u>to help</u>

her and I was <u>trying to row</u> us back. The (storm) got worse,

with (lightning) and thunder. (Huge waves) nearly <u>capsized</u>

us. (I woke up in a sweat. The dream was so real I had to

check to see if Janet was okay. She's in her sixth month

and everything is fine, but that dream really shook me up!)

Eric felt that all the words he circled (Janet, I, rowboat, lake, sunny day, oars, darkened sky, belly, baby, shore, storm, lightning, thunder, huge waves) represented the pregnancy, especially the "sunny day." He thought the storm with its darkened sky, thunder, lightning, and huge waves symbolized his perception of the way labor and delivery were going to be.

Eric diagrammed the action or plot of his dream by underlining these words: taking turns, began to rain, clutching, yelling, was coming, tried not to panic, screaming, to help, trying to row, capsized. This enabled him to see the meaning of his dream.

As the lake changed from a peaceful place into a storm-ravaged, dangerous environment, it became obvious to Eric that this indeed was a labor scene, with Janet yelling that the baby was coming. "At first we were sharing, taking turns with the oars. Then all of a sudden it was up to me," he said, "and I couldn't handle it." Eric thought his comments—"I tried not to panic" and "I woke up in a sweat"—indicated a loss of control over the situation, as the boat (symbolizing Janet's pregnancy) was about to capsize due to the high waves (labor contractions). An inexperienced expectant father, Eric clearly was worried that he might not be able to provide the support and morale-boosting his wife would need from him when she went into labor.

Now, let's take a look at Janet's dream and the way she diagrammed it:

In this dream I am <u>floating</u> on my back in a swimming pool on a large cruise ship. The water is warm and I <u>feel very happy</u> because the water sort of <u>buoys me up</u>. My stomach is <u>looming over</u> me because I am <u>very pregnant</u>. I am so big, I <u>can't see</u> my toes. But I <u>feel safe</u> because everything <u>is very calm</u>. Then I notice all the other swimmers are also pregnant. I notice the lifeguard and realize it is Eric. Then alarm bells and sirens <u>start</u> up, making a horrible, deafening noise. At first I think it is a drill but the sky gets black, icy raindrops hit my skin, and the ship <u>begins</u> to roll. Big waves <u>rise up</u> in the pool. Some of the women <u>start screaming</u> and <u>trying to get out</u>. But I <u>can't move.</u> I <u>try to turn over</u> but my stomach is too heavy. I <u>try to kick</u> but <u>can't feel</u> anything. I get a mouthful of water and <u>start to choke</u>. Eric <u>throws</u> in a ring but I <u>can't reach</u> it. I <u>realize</u> he <u>is too busy</u> with everyone <u>screaming</u> and <u>milling</u>

around and that(he) can't help (me) (At this point I woke

up, feeling terrified.)

Janet circled this dream's many water symbols (swimming pool, cruise ship, warm water, other pregnant swimmers, lifeguard, raindrops, big waves, mouthful of water), indicating her pregnancy. The direct reference to pregnancy is almost as if her dreaming self wanted to make sure that she didn't miss the symbolism.

Janet thought the other pregnant women in the pool symbolized the Lamaze class that she and Eric had just begun attending. When we discussed these dreams Janet admitted to a slight jealousy of some of the other women in the class, who she thought were more attractive because "they're not as huge as I am." These feelings may account for her fear at the end of the dream that the lifeguard (Eric) is too busy helping everybody else to rescue her.

Then Janet underlined all these action words: floating, feel very happy, buoys me up, looming over, can't see, (sirens) start, (sky) gets black, (ship) begins to roll, (waves) rise up, start screaming, trying to get out, can't move, try to turn over, try to kick, can't feel, start to choke, (Eric) throws, can't reach, (Eric) is too busy, (everyone) screaming, milling around, I realize (he) can't help.

Like the lake of Eric's dream, Janet's swimming pool became a dangerous and chaotic place in the midst of a sudden storm. Again, huge waves (symbolizing the onset of labor) nearly drowned her. She lost control of her body and awakened terrified when she realized her husband could not help her.

As we discussed her fears, Janet began to view much of her panic and worry as needless. She also understood that by using Lamaze techniques—relaxing and "flowing with" the wavelike feelings of labor contractions—she would in fact be able to control them.

Janet and Eric continued learning about the details of

labor and delivery in their Lamaze classes, and their night-marish dreams subsided. The father-to-be came through brilliantly, giving Janet constant support and coaching during her eight-hour labor. He was the first to hold their baby girl and to put her into Janet's arms.

To get more practice in diagramming, let's assess two dreams from Penny, a 28-year-old marketing consultant for a dress manufacturer. In early pregnancy, Penny recorded this dream:

> I'm at the hospital where I used to work, feeling happy. In my dream I have the same job. The staff doesn't seem busy that day so several of us are repotting bulbs. I have a big, round planter box in front of me but can't finish the project, as I got the soil too wet and have to wait for it to dry. I feel very impatient and keep looking at the calendar, hoping I can get the bulbs planted and growing well before August.

Without looking at my diagram of Penny's dream, try your hand at it. Later, you can compare your results with mine. Now, diagram the dream Penny submitted in her sixth month:

> I'm setting up a high-fashion design group with several
>
> others (my actual job, which I just left on maternity
>
> leave). At some point I sleep with the owner and it is okay
>
> because I'm not married in the dream. Then he and I have
>
> a misunderstanding but I transfer. I plan to move to the
>
> Southwest. Three retired men who used to work at my old
>
> office at the hospital appear and congratulate me on my
>
> new position and they hint that I am getting out of a

sticky situation. I return to the main office and see that the owner and a beautiful brunette woman are now lovers. I awake feeling very jealous and upset and then realize the boss in my dream looked like my husband. (All night after this dream I wasn't able to sleep because I kept wondering if my husband is actually having an affair.)

Here is the way I diagrammed Penny's first dream:

I'm at the hospital where I used to work. In my dream I have the same job. The staff doesn't seem busy that day so several of us are repotting bulbs. I have a big round planter box in front of me but can't finish the project, as I got the soil too wet and have to wait for it to dry. I feel very impatient and keep looking at the calendar, hoping I can get the bulbs planted and growing well before August.

Penny was one of the volunteers in my doctoral research project, so she had not yet learned to diagram her dreams. However, she thought the words that I circled symbolized her early pregnancy: bulbs (growing things yet to reach full flowering), the big round planter box (her womb), and the wet soil (indicating fertility). Penny's feelings of impatience were also typical of this period, because she was awaiting delivery with great anticipation. Her due date was not until August, a fact clearly indicated in her dream.

Also notice that both of Penny's dreams took place in office settings. This may hint at something important about Penny's concerns. This is the way I diagrammed her later dream:

(I'm) setting up a (high-fashion) design (group) with several

others (my actual job, which I just left on maternity

leave). At some point (I) sleep with the (owner) and it is okay

because (I'm) not married in the dream. Then (he) and (I) have

a misunderstanding but (I) transfer. (I) plan to move to the

Southwest. Three retired (men who) used to work at my old

(office) at the (hospital) appear and congratulate (me) on my

(new position) and they hint that (I) am getting out of a

(sticky situation.) (I) return to the main (office) and see that the

owner and a beautiful brunette (woman) are now lovers. (I)

awake feeling very jealous and upset and then realize the

(boss) in my dream looked like my (husband.) (All night after

this dream I wasn't able to sleep because I kept wondering

if my husband is actually having an affair.)

When Penny described her job in our interview, she commented, "I was beginning to feel out of place there, because I'm so pregnant now. I just felt conspicuous with all these showroom models gliding around, so I was relieved to go on maternity leave." The main symbols and verbs in her dream indicate that Penny surely was glad to "get out of a sticky situation." At the same time, she worried about not fitting in when she returned. "I plan to take the baby to work," she explained, "and that's okay with my boss. That way I can nurse, but now I think I may feel even more out of place than I do now."

Obviously, Penny was more deeply upset by her changing appearance than she admitted to herself, since her dream also indicated that she feared the loss of her husband to another woman. It's also possible that Penny was concerned that someone else might take over her job while she was having the baby. As it turned out, Penny's husband remained perfectly faithful and she gave birth to a normal baby girl. She decided not to return to work and reported great satisfaction with being a full-time homemaker.

Practicing Step 2

Having practiced interpreting Hazel, Janet, Eric, and Penny's dreams, it's time to try your skills on your own. First reread your dream diary. Then, remembering that a dream symbol is usually *an image or picture that stands for something else,* circle all the words that are symbols in your dreams. These will include characters (people, animals), objects, and settings.

Now write down your associations to these words. What do they remind you of in your waking life? In this way, you can discover how your symbols match or seem different from the list of typical pregnancy dream symbols. Imagine that you are describing these dream elements to someone who knows nothing at all about them.

Better yet, practice with your partner or a friend. Frequently, just sharing your dream aloud will give you a more objective view of it. Have your partner or friend question you about the dream symbols you have circled and describe your associations for each one.

When the correct meaning of a symbol comes to mind, you should get an "aha!" feeling, a conviction of hitting upon the right interpretation. This chapter's categorization of dream symbols may be helpful as well. Or you may decide your symbols have an entirely different meaning.

Next, examine the action and the plot of your dream. Underline all the verbs in your dream description. Does the action in your dream remind you of anything going on in your waking life?

Try to describe the plot of your dream in one or two short sentences. For example, Penny might say about her first dream, "I am happily busy, planting bulbs in a large container. Then I get impatient because the soil isn't ready and I have to wait. I'm hoping the bulbs will bloom by August."

Now that you've described the action or plot of your own dream, you should be well on the way to interpreting it and seeing more clearly whether or not you've repressed some fears or worries. Or perhaps you'll discover a conflict or problem in your waking life that needs to be addressed before you can minimize stress.

Some readers may be able to identify the feelings without knowing why they occurred. A better understanding of your emotions will also help you learn to use your daydreams as well as your dreams to relieve the worries and anxieties that could be preventing you from enjoying a relaxed and joyful pregnancy.

❖

Step 3: Understanding Your Emotions

Tammy, a 23-year-old fashion model, had this dream in her third month:

> I'm posing in an evening gown for a very famous photographer (I'm not pregnant in the dream). It's going to be a magazine cover. The photographer says, "You have a long chin. Drop it a little and let's have a smile." So I just take hold of my chin, and it comes right off in my hand! In the dream, this seems perfectly normal. I hide the chin in the folds of the evening dress and smile. But I don't feel like smiling at all. I feel like crying. Then the photographer stops to fix the lights and I take some tear shaped crystals

out of my eyes and hide those too. He comes back. "What did you do to your eyes?" he says. "They look dull, not shiny like before." And I yell at him, "What do you want from me, anyhow?" and I throw the chin and the tears in his face. (Then I woke up.)

After we diagrammed her dream, Tammy thought it reflected her worries about sudden, uncontrollable emotions. "I'm not showing yet, so I can still work awhile," she explained. "But I never can be sure how I might react. The least little thing may set me off to either crying or getting mad. In my business, I can't afford that. Before I got pregnant, I was always able to hide my feelings and turn on the smiles, even when I felt sad." Tammy had chosen a career where she could use her ability to repress her emotions to advantage, at least until she became pregnant. Then she confided, "One thing I'll never do is to make my child hide her feelings the way I was taught. The truth is, it really feels good nowadays to have an excuse to cry when my feelings get hurt."

However, Tammy's inability to control her emotions during pregnancy proved to be a blessing in disguise. The reason it felt good when she expressed herself by crying was that Tammy was allowing her mind and body to react normally. After a lifetime of repressing her true feelings, Tammy's pregnancy forced her to release her emotions.

One of the major producers of stress is the repression of emotions. Dr. Stephen Polsky, a psychologist in Walnut Creek, California, points out that repressed emotions ultimately may come out in a different form. For instance, concealed anger sometimes manifests itself as depression or actual symptoms of physical disease, such as the high blood pressure, nausea, and headaches that many pregnant women experience. Emotional expression need not be inappropriate. If you are like Tammy and have not been able to let others know your true feelings in the past, this is an ideal time to begin, because pregnancy naturally evokes intense and varied emotions. You also may find yourself unable to hide the strong emotions that just pour out despite your efforts to control them.

There are several reasons for the unusual state of your emotions during pregnancy, specifically hormonal, physical, and psychological changes.

Physical Changes

Early pregnancy. During the first three or four months, the rapid increase in your body's hormones will probably result in sudden mood shifts, from outbursts of tears to unexplainable displays of anger. These emotional explosions may happen anywhere—at home, in your office, on the street—and the person who happens to be your "target" may quite naturally be puzzled or hurt. This chapter shows you several ways to safely release emotions so that you can express yourself appropriately without having to conceal these feelings.

Dr. Sheila Kitzinger explains that levels of the hormones *estrogen* and *progesterone* increase dramatically and remain at higher levels throughout your pregnancy. Nature's purpose here is to build up the lining of the uterus, providing a protective, nutritious environment for your baby to develop.

Unfortunately, the new mother's emotional equilibrium frequently suffers as a result of this process. Recent medical studies in Great Britain and Scandinavia indicate that high levels of estrogen speed up the body's production of *tryptophan*. This amino acid is necessary for the body's production of *serotonin,* an important chemical that helps prevent depression. Therefore, the sudden increase in estrogen during pregnancy inhibits your body's usual biochemical methods of stress avoidance.

Just as imbalance between the two hormones estrogen and progesterone prior to a menstrual period contributes to the tensions associated with Premenstrual Syndrome (PMS), so does this temporary imbalance cause extreme mood swings in many newly pregnant women. Additionally, many have the swollen, tender breasts and water retention also typical of PMS.

These emotions may remind you of the feelings you endured during your teens. Then, as now, you possibly felt self-conscious and awkward about your rapidly changing body and overloaded with many see-saw moods and emotions. Maybe you found—and will find—relief in a sudden burst of tears or a display of temper.

Some expectant mothers also have "hot flashes" similar to those reported by menopausal women. All of these symptoms result from shifts in hormone levels. None of this is comfortable; most of it, in fact, is distressing. However, you should take heart from the fact that your hormone levels will soon achieve a balance lasting until delivery.

Late pregnancy changes. Even after your hormones are balanced, both estrogen and progesterone appear at high levels. Therefore, expect that your emotions and all your senses will continue to be more intense and varied than before you conceived. Also as your pregnancy progresses, you probably will become even more uncomfortable physically, especially in the eighth month. Decreased mobility and the pressures of the uterus may give you an embarrassingly leaky bladder.

It's natural for you to be impatient and anxious at this time. Again, let optimism prevail: the baby soon will "engage" or drop down into your pelvis, making it a bit easier for you to carry.

Postpartum emotional states. The physical changes and resulting emotional intensity of pregnancy usually subside after the baby is born. Women who do not wish to nurse are given medications that prevent the milk from coming in. This may contribute to postpartum depression; recent studies show that the inhibition of *prolactin,* the hormone producing breast milk, affects emotional stability. Therefore, some women—especially those who do not nurse—experience either a strong lack of emotion or a depression (called the "after baby blues"). One way to avoid this condition is to allow your milk to come in naturally.

Psychological Changes

Following her in-depth study in 1980, Dr. Myra Leifer concluded that even women who had a strong sense of self-esteem prior to pregnancy suffered from severe anxiety and lack of confidence in their ability to mother. My own research in 1986 showed even more widespread fears. The emotional turmoil caused by hormonal changes is exacerbated by other external and psychological factors.

While intertwined with physical variables, the emotional upheavals of pregnancy also arise from a transition demanding greater responsibility and maturity. Most people exhibit signs of turmoil and stress during life's transitional stages. One major maturational crisis is adolescence. The next transition occurs as you become an adult. Now, as an expectant mother, you are in the midst of making the final leap to maturity.

Many expectant females may not have resolved all the problems of adolescence. Tension surfaces when they try to move directly from girlhood to motherhood without having first fully accepted the responsibilities of womanhood.

One easy way to find out whether you are still in conflict about adolescent issues is to examine your dreams. If they frequently depict your past and your parents—especially your mother—you probably have some unresolved problems going back to your teenage years. Many pregnant women's dreams, for example, portray their mothers as disapproving authority figures.

If you confront these issues, you can better assume your rightful role as an adult. Childbirth researcher Tracy Hotchner says that emotional growth occurs when women resolve the confusion of pregnancy. Hotchner also points out that expectant mothers soon realize that almost every area of their lives are being affected by their condition. Your relationship with your mate, your adequacy as a person and a mother-to-be, your mortality, even your views on world peace—all these and more assume added significance in your mind.

For example, in her seventh month, 34-year-old Meryl had this dream:

> Dreamed my stomach had turned into a globe of the world. The equator ran right around my belly button! As I looked at it closely, I could see little eruptions happening in Europe and Asia. Then a tiny bullet rose out of Russia and landed on America. At the same time, another bullet came out of Washington, D.C. headed toward Russia. The tiny explosions were very painful and then my whole stomach burst into flames (and I woke up screaming).

We can clearly see that Meryl's concern about the state of the world was connected to her perceptions of pregnancy and her unborn child's fate. Such worries naturally evolve from interest in your baby's future and, while the intensity of this kind of anxiety may be surprising, it is not abnormal.

According to Dr. Ernest Hartmann, many people report an increase in the frequency of their nightmares during transitional times. Since our dreams consistently reflect the conflicts and problems of our waking life, it's not surprising that most pregnancy dreams are filled with turmoil and images of fear and loss. Researchers tell us we should welcome these nightmares because they call our attention to a conflict or problem we may have been avoiding and to the accompanying repressed emotions. Dr. Theodore Isaac Rubin, a psychiatrist well-known for his studies of anger, calls these repressed emotions our "slush fund," a literal pool of toxins and poisons draining into our bodies.

Dream researcher and psychologist Patricia Garfield urges us to see nightmares as important and meaningful, and then to engage in activities and thoughts that will ease the anxiety. She cites studies of children who suffered frequent bad dreams. When encouraged to participate in activities directly related to their fears, these young people ceased to have nightmares. My own experience with pregnant women confirms Dr. Garfield's general findings.

Identifying the Emotions of Pregnancy Dreams

During a recent interview focusing on my work as a pregnancy psychologist, the reporter (whom I'll call Pamela) suddenly blurted out, "You know, one reason I'm so interested in this assignment is that I'm two months pregnant, and I'm about at my wit's end. I'm hoping you can give me some advice about my own nightmares."

When I asked Pamela to describe one of her recent nightmares, she told me:

I dreamed my husband and I were on the roof of a narrow skyscraper. He wanted me to walk on this small, flimsy plank across to the next building. He gave me an armful of packages and bags of groceries to carry. I said I couldn't possibly get across and juggle all these bundles at the same time. I felt upset that he expected this. He just left me there and went on across. He waved and told me it was easy, to hurry up and cross on the plank. There were a lot of (women) over there with him. At least a dozen. I couldn't tell who they were. (He) shouted that (everybody) else could cross on that plank and that (I) was chicken (I) looked down and dropped some of the (bags) of groceries. There were some kind of (ugly little animals) like (mice) or (rats) in them, which fell out and splattered onto the street below (I) felt very scared but determined to try. I stepped onto the plank and felt dizzy and sick. (That's all I remember except I woke up feeling nauseated and had to run to the bathroom fast before I threw up.)

You may want to try your new skills in understanding dream symbols to make sense of Pamela's nightmare. From the highlighted words, we can see how her journey from one building to another possibly represented pregnancy. Clearly, she perceived this supposedly blissful period as one fraught with danger and potential harm.

The physical tension resulting from unexpressed emotions sometimes results in unhealthy side effects. Pamela may have been experiencing this, because she complained of frequent headaches, nausea, and depression. "But if I can't even recognize my emotions when I'm having them," Pamela wondered, "then how can I possibly express them?" I explained that first she must understand the reasons she was repressing or blocking her emotions. With this accomplished, Pamela would be able to explore a variety of techniques that could help her express herself more openly.

BLOCKS TO EXPRESSING EMOTIONS

Some of the typical blocks to emotional expression are misconceptions about the "negativity" of emotions; fear of loss of control; and fear of disapproval. When we talked about emotions, Pamela showed difficulty identifying "negative" feelings, such as anger and pain. Rubin explains that many parents take a double-bind position, telling their children to release anger, fear, or pain, but punishing them for being disrespectful when they express such feelings.

Psychiatrist Daniel Casriel, in *A Scream Away From Happiness,* comments that girls are told to repress anger more often than boys. Even in today's so-called liberated culture, females who express anger openly may be considered unfeminine and too aggressive. Many women consequently spend their lives secretly believing that they are bad or somehow abnormal because they harbor angry feelings.

Further, women often think anger, fear, and pain indicate instability or a lack of control. If anyone—especially their mates, close friends, and doctors—suspected them of such emotions, the women would be judged poor parents. Or perhaps a lack of mental and emotional control points to insanity. Could they possibly pass this on to their unborn children?

In 1975, Dr. S. A. Arbeit of Yale University reported that the pregnant women in her study exhibited this type of denial, despite evidence of stress symptoms. The volunteers in my 1986 doctoral research also frequently refused to admit to any of the anger and fear reflected in their dreams. Finally, Van de Castle noted that most pregnant women appear reluctant to discuss the terrifying nature of their nightmares, "lest it be thought that they must really resent their pregnancy. Statistically it is far more common to experience these intense anxiety dreams in pregnancy."

As a result of denial and repression, some women begin to believe they have no stress, even though their dreams and waking states provide strong evidence to the contrary. If you wish to break this pattern, you must understand that, like most women, you probably have been inhibited from recognizing or responding to your emotions. Acceptance of all your feelings as normal and natural will help you confront the issues your dreams reflect.

While most nightmares portray fear and terror, at least a hint of another emotion or feeling usually surfaces. For instance, Pamela mentioned that she was "upset" with her husband for compelling her to walk the plank depicted in her dreams. When I asked her if she ever expressed anger toward him, Pamela gave me a puzzled look. "But I'm not angry with him," she insisted. "We hardly ever disagree. Oh, I did feel a little annoyed with him in that dream, when he kept insisting I juggle all those bags and try to walk across that dangerous place. But I'm not really angry with him, not when I'm awake."

With a few gentle prods from me, Pamela finally admitted to a number of things causing her increased resentment toward her husband. Although she had agreed it was time for them to become parents, she derived much satisfaction from her work as a journalist for a large city newspaper. Pamela also felt her husband unsympathetic about the many physical changes she was experiencing and about her fears of being unable to continue her promising career. "I do *want* this baby," she said, "but sometimes I actually wish I'd have a miscarriage."

In *The Experience of Childbirth,* Kitzinger points out that many newly pregnant women are not emotionally prepared for their new roles and may be filled with self-deprecation because they believe they should be blissfully happy about their condition. This ambivalence is not new: expectant mothers have suffered from these conflicts for decades. However, today's woman may be feeling them more intensely because of the Superwoman Syndrome, the need to appear perfect, as discussed in Chapter 1. Fortunately for both mother and baby, the conflict is usually resolved as the mother accepts her pregnancy, a process Dr. Helene Deutsch calls psychological "incorporation of the fetus." This usually happens by the third trimester.

Once Pamela understood that she was entitled to have and express all her feelings, she began to examine some of the attitudes previously blocking her awareness of them. It's no easy task to undo a lifetime of conditioning. Yet pregnant women possess one major advantage: intensified emotions. As Tammy the fashion model commented, "It used to be a lot easier to ignore feeling a little mad or a bit sad. Now, every feeling is so big, there's really no way to avoid it."

Once you stop categorizing emotions as either good or bad, you will view them as a natural protection mechanism and safety valve.

THE BASIC EMOTIONS

To identify your feelings, you need only learn about four basic emotions: anger, fear, pain, and pleasure and love. While each of these emotions has many degrees—such as happiness, annoyance, caution, and sadness—understanding the fundamentals will help you identify the other various degrees of emotions.

In identifying the basic emotions, I've found the following procedure to be the most effective: first sound it out; then name your emotion; finally, notice the body clues and physical sensations.

The easiest way to pinpoint your feelings is to make a sound. Do this when you've had an upsetting nightmare and cannot understand it, or you can practice at any other convenient time, day or night.

Simply take a deep breath and then shout, yell, sigh, groan, or moan. Or, after inhaling and exhaling slowly to relax your vocal chords, catch another breath and say "Ahhhhhh" or "Ohhhhhh" as loudly as possible. (You will need a private place to try this. Some of my clients even get in their cars and roll up the windows to be sure no one hears them.) Don't be surprised when you experience immediate, strong body sensations such as sudden tears or perhaps the intense energy associated with anger.

While this process may seem ridiculous at first, scientific evidence suggests a linkage between sounds and emotions. Dr. William Fry, Jr., a biochemist in the psychiatry department of the St. Paul-Ramsey Medical Center, has conducted studies indicating that toxic substances build up in the body when painful emotions are not released. Fry further noticed that moaning, groaning, and crying help release these poisons and restore the body's normal balance. The natural, healthy way to express emotions, therefore, is to make sounds.

I also applaud Dr. Daniel Casriel's techniques because they can be adapted to situations outside the therapist's office. To practice identifying and expressing your emotions using his methods, all you usually need to do is make sounds. This brings immediate relief and recognition of repressed emotions.

Dr. Louis Savory, clinical psychologist and dream researcher, asks clients to stretch out on the carpet and groan loudly. He says this simple process is one of the most effective ways to deal with tension and stress. Savory also encourages clients to keep their car windows rolled up and groan away the day's pressures as they drive home from work.

After you have made a sound, take special notice of the resulting physical signals and then name the emotion. Say, either aloud or to yourself, "I'm feeling (anger, fear, pain, or pleasure)." Just articulate whatever emotion popped into your head as you made the sound.

Many pregnant women find this simple technique extremely effective in pinpointing their feelings. For example, when Tammy the fashion model made a very loud "Ahhhhhh" sound, she said, "Wow! That sounds like I'm mad!" After I suggested she substitute "angry" for "mad," Tammy released another hearty "Ahhhhhh," followed with "I'm angry!" Some tears rolled down Tammy's cheeks and she brushed them away impatiently. "That's just memories of my parents telling me it isn't nice to be angry," she said. With our encouragement, Tammy then stood up and informed each one of us, in a very loud voice, "I'm angry and it's okay!" After doing this a dozen times, she and the entire group shouted "I'm angry!" and laughed with relief. Then Tammy told us, "The main reason I'm angry is that I'm tired of holding in my feelings, and I'm not going to do it any longer."

After her healthy baby girl was born, Tammy called me to report a career change from modeling to acting. "I'll never return to being that frozen, smiling model," she said. "Emotional expression is important in acting, and I'm ready for it. Already I've been offered my first part, after only one audition."

Although none of my other students made such dramatic career changes, by simply "sounding it out" they soon learned to recognize the repressed emotions that surfaced in their nightmares. They also compared dreamed feelings with waking ones.

For example, when 32-year-old Jill, a successful real estate agent in her sixth month, practiced making sounds, she discovered fear. Her "Ahhhhhh" came out more like a call for help than an angry outburst. After Jill put her head on another student's shoulder and tried some moaning sounds, she told us, "All my noises sound like a scared little girl, so I must be feeling fear." We then asked for possible reasons. The only one Jill could think of was that she sometimes became "a little nervous" when showing a prospective client property.

The next week, Jill reported this dream:

> Dreamed I was showing some property to a woman who looked like my mother. She had four little children, from an infant to an eight-year-old, and she asked me to take care of the baby and the next older one—he was still in diapers—in the car, while she and the other kids looked at the house. The minute she got out of the car, both

babies started crying. She looked back and said, "I know you can handle this. After all, you're a mother now, yourself." And I tried to look competent, but I was scared. I started changing the little baby and then the other one began pointing to his pants and crying, letting me know he needed changing, too. Stuck myself with the diaper pin and my blood was pouring out. Couldn't move either one of my arms. The bigger baby was crawling around and somehow released the brake and the car started to roll. Out the window, I could see my client and her other two kids coming, looking surprised and angry. (I woke up feeling upset and wondering how I'll ever be able to manage.)

Jill told us that this dream not only indicated her fear of being a failure as a mother (trying to look competent and feeling scared), but also reflected her worries about parental disapproval (the maternal client looking surprised and angry), and the task of balancing career and children (wondering how she would ever be able to manage).

Still, many pregnant women have been accustomed to ignoring or repressing their emotions for so long that even screaming or moaning doesn't help. When Pamela, the distressed reporter, tried making sounds, she immediately began to exhibit body language associated with a mixture of pain and anger. Her face became flushed, she breathed more rapidly, and tears welled up in her eyes.

When I asked, "What are you feeling?" she could only shake her head and reply, "Just, well, very upset." Then I said, "Don't be embarrassed. It's all right to cry if you feel like it." Pamela's response was to sob. As we talked, it became obvious that she could allow herself to cry and admit she might be feeling pain. However, like many women, her attitudes about anger blocked her expression of that emotion.

To overcome attitudinal blocks, it helps to know the physical signs of each emotion. When I explained to Pamela that her rapid breathing, accelerated heartbeat, and flushed face might indicate anger, she confessed to having some resentments about her pregnancy and her husband's seeming lack of support.

The chart on page 116 was derived from the work of Dr. Casriel, a psychiatrist who helped found the system of emotional re-education based on the connections between sounds and feelings. It is designed to help you match your physical signs with the appropriate emotions. Each of the basic emotions listed in the chart possesses specific attributes:

Anger. Anger is the general term applied to many degrees of displeasure, some of which appear in parentheses on the chart.

When any stimulus, either physical or mental, real or imagined, makes us angry, adrenalin rushes into the blood, affecting the circulatory system and causing the heart to beat faster. Extra blood leaves the skin and other organs and surges to the brain and muscles. Our bodies produce more red blood corpuscles, so the blood clots faster and its pressure rises.

Digestion also comes to an abrupt halt, reducing stomach and intestinal movement and the secretion of gastric juices. If we have just eaten or are in the process of doing so, anger may cause indigestion or nausea. The rectum and bladder don't empty easily when we're angry. Carbohydrates stored in the liver enter our bloodstreams, giving added sugar; therefore, we feel stronger and more energetic. Breathing gets faster and deeper. Our hair literally stands on end, and we tend to sweat or perspire more freely.

Nature gave us these responses to prepare us for self-defense. When we are angry, the extra blood in our brains and muscles allows us to make quick decisions and take strenuous action. In fact, all the bodily changes listed above fortify us in dangerous situations.

When we do not express ourselves and instead repress anger, these physical changes have no outlet and make us

Matching Physical Signs to Appropriate Emotions

Emotion	Physical Signs	Healthy Attitude
Anger (rage, fury, indignation, wrath, ire, resentment, frustration, annoyance)	Increased heart rate and blood pressure; rapid, deep breathing; indigestion; flushed face; erect hair; muscle strength; increased brain activity (speeded-up thoughts).	I am entitled to all my feelings. I'm good enough. I count. I'm me.
Fear (terror, fright, panic, alarm, dread, anxiety, nervousness)	Increased heart rate; lower blood pressure; slower brain activity; loss of bladder and bowel control; pale face; cool or clammy sweat; rapid, shallow breathing.	I'm afraid and it's okay. I need help and that's all right. If I make mistakes, I can start over again.
Pain (agony, suffering, hurt feelings, sorrow, grief, distress)	Muscle tension; abdominal, pelvic, and groin spasms; blurred vision; tears; dizziness; ragged breathing; irregular heart rate, blood pressure and temperature, and other symptoms of shock, incoherent speech	I'm hurting. I need help. I need love. My feelings are beautiful. I'm lovable.
Pleasure and love (happiness, contentment, joy, desire, passion)	Relaxed muscles; steady, even breathing; absence of tension; smiles; giggles; sexual arousal; overall well-being.	I am lovable, and my feelings are normal. I can control my emotions. I am huggable, desirable.

feel bad. Society now demands that we control aggressive emotions, yet our bodies continue to prepare us for defending against danger, just as they did fifty thousand years ago. Repressed feelings may well be one of the major causes of stress in modern times. Consider also that the chemical changes taking place in a pregnant woman's body pass to the fetus through the placenta. This makes it even more important for expectant mothers to release anger. Some natural outlets are: shouting, screaming, and yelling; physically attacking; and communicating angry feelings to the person who hurt us.

Unlike our ancestors who faced physical dangers (wild animals, attacking tribes of other humans), we usually cannot defend ourselves with violent methods. Certainly it's seldom permissible to scream or yell, unless at a sports event. However, you can roll up those car windows or find other safe places to release anger when the pressure builds. Once the extreme emotional charge is diffused, you can speak out about your feelings. In fact, most pregnant women who assert themselves immediately usually find that their anger rarely builds to the point where they need to shout and yell.

Fear. Fear is a strong, usually unpleasant emotion arising out of danger or the anticipation of it. Some of the degrees of fear are listed in parentheses on the chart. While provoking some of the same physical changes experienced during anger, fear presents major differences, specifically decreased brain activity.

All of us are familiar with the effects of panic. When we are "scared out of our minds" (the saying is literally true), blood circulates away from the brain, so that we may "go blank" for a few moments. Adrenalin pours into the bloodstream as in anger, and the heart pumps more rapidly. Our muscles also grow stronger. With no distracting thoughts, with additional adrenalin, and with stronger muscles, our threatened ancestors probably escaped from danger without taking time to think about it. Today, it's usually unrealistic or impossible to run away from danger this quickly. Nevertheless, your body continues to prepare you for flight; if you don't somehow express the fear, you may encounter all the ill effects of stress and anxiety discussed in Chapter 1.

Other physical effects of fear include shortness of breath, damp palms, and sweating. Some stage-frightened actresses actually experience convulsive stomach pains or succumb to fainting. During fearful moments, the digestive system reacts opposite to the way it does during anger; we tend to lose control of digestive functions. Since pregnant women already are more prone to these problems, the additional burden of unexpressed fear proves particularly troublesome.

The natural outlets of fear are screaming, whimpering, and crying or sobbing. Of course, it's often unacceptable to express yourself in these ways, but sometimes the situation improves merely by admitting that you're afraid. Or you can roll up those car windows again and let go with a real horror movie-type of scream—a wonderful release for fear as well as anger.

Pain. Pain is an unpleasant sensation due to bodily or mental injury. Its degrees (shown in parentheses on the chart) can range from intense, sometimes unbearable agony to milder levels of distress.

The bodily changes accompanying emotional and physical pain are similar. These include muscle tension and spasms (especially in the abdomen, pelvis, and groin), a sore or aching throat, blurred vision, and dizziness.

When we hold back emotional pain, muscle tension and spasms increase. The biochemist Dr. William Fry tells us that tears cleanse us of toxins. Women normally have sixty percent more of the hormone *prolactin* in their bloodstreams than men. Since prolactin stimulates the tear glands, this may account for the fact that women cry more easily. Interestingly, prolactin levels increase as the pregnancy progresses, possibly intensifying emotions further. When tears are not released, toxins may clog the sinuses and cause searing physical pain in the ears and throat. Additionally, fear sometimes arises from our emotion-blocking attitudes about pain. The body's burden increases, as the symptoms of both fear and pain may appear. Finally, the physical changes accompanying both pain and fear also occur with the repression of emotional distress. The harmful effects on a pregnant woman's body—and therefore upon the unborn child—are doubled as well.

The natural outlets for emotional pain include crying and weeping, moaning and groaning, and sobbing.

When you feel sad and cannot cry, try Dr. Gay Gaer Luce's technique. In *Your Second Life,* she suggests putting your hand on the upper part of your chest, near the collarbone, and then starting to breathe only as deeply as possible without causing your hand to move. Once you've established this shallow breathing pattern, make a sound like a crying baby. Listen to yourself, noticing the sad tone. Think of what has been causing pain in your life recently and continue to make sobbing sounds. Deliberately wallow in self-pity. Let the tears flow and your muscle tension ease. The relief you will experience is true relaxation.

Pleasure and love. Some psychiatrists and psychologists consider these agreeable emotions as one and the same. Pleasure is described by Dr. Casriel as the feeling of having one's needs met by others and by one's self. According to his definition, love means the anticipation of pleasure, both through our relationships with others and from our own self-esteem. (Some of the other degrees of pleasure and love are listed in parentheses on the chart of emotions.)

For centuries, poets and songwriters have extolled the physical effects of romantic love—feelings of elation and bliss so intense it leaves one giddy, intoxicated. By making us eager to touch and be touched, to give and accept sexual pleasures with the loved one, nature may be preparing us to conceive.

The expectant mother's normal desires often increase because of the rise in her hormone levels. Furthermore, the breasts and genital tissues are engorged with extra blood, and vaginal lubrication accelerates.

Childbirth researcher Hotchner comments that many pregnant women become an embodiment of the "Earth Mother," with a heavier scent and extra lubrication. Some appear highly erotic and experience unusual sexual fantasies. This sudden surge of sensuality may be overwhelming to their mates. If this happens to you, give your partner a little time to adjust.

The sudden change to ultrafemininity also frightens many expectant mothers. Those with previously low sex drive may feel even more overwhelmed than their partners. If a sudden increase in your erotic desires bothers you, it's most important to discuss it with your mate. He may feel equally overwhelmed. Simply letting him know your feelings will reduce both of your fears.

If these sexual needs are unfulfilled, however, the effects on your body may simulate those caused by repressed anger. When any woman, pregnant or not, finds her desires ignored or unnoticed, she's likely to feel rejected or, at the least, very touchy and irritable. This makes it all the more important for her to share her feelings and thoughts with her mate.

The release of tension and the bonded closeness coming from intimacy is beneficial to the pregnant woman's physical state. Moreover, her mate's caresses help to dispel any self-doubts about her desirability. These delightful feelings also cause bodily changes, such as increased endorphin levels and a strengthened immune system, which are transmitted to the fetus through the mother's bloodstream.

Some couples fear that intercourse may endanger the unborn child. This rarely holds true, provided some precautions are taken to ensure the woman's comfort. During the third trimester, those who find intercourse uncomfortable or even painful may learn to achieve orgasm solely with the caresses formerly reserved for foreplay. The woman in late pregnancy can also explore new ways to satisfy her mate, such as stroking and kissing him all over his body. Surprisingly, pleasure also immediately results from expressing anger, fear, or emotional pain. One of the first rewards may be a feeling of relief and an absence of tension, due to the relaxation of previously strained muscles.

Indeed, when we express our emotions openly, we realize at a very deep, psychological level that we can face and deal with almost anything. Renewed strength and courage then add to our feelings of pleasure.

For instance, Pamela, the reporter whose pregnant feelings were in such turmoil, finally identified and dealt with her resentments. She later called to tell me this good news: "All I had to do was to let my husband know my misgivings about being able to have a baby and keep my career. Once I told him about how some of his tactless remarks hurt me, he apologized. Since then, things are a lot easier. Now, the future looks brighter." Pamela's articles about my work and her own emotional struggles helped many women—so much so that a local hospital invited her to lead a support group for expectant mothers.

The natural outlets of pleasure and love include giggles, smiles, and laughter; sighs and touching; and sexual arousal and orgasm.

Healthy Emotional Attitudes

Expectant women who, like my reporter friend Pamela, experienced frightening or depressed periods early in pregnancy may have difficulty in allowing themselves to feel the happiness of the moment. Just as positive thoughts can produce upbeat feelings, dwelling on the negative can perpetuate anxiety or fear.

To test this idea, try thinking about your favorite food. Notice the saliva in your mouth flowing. Now, feel the puckering as you imagine the taste of a lemon. In a similar fashion, our thoughts can evoke more extreme physical states. If we concentrate on dismal or fearful possibilities, bodily changes may impel us to highly negative actions. These habits or patterns of thought generally stem from attitudes developed since childhood.

To help yourself change these attitudes, remember that all of our emotions and feelings are normal. Accept and express them fully and you can avoid the ill effects of stress.

EMOTIONAL EXPRESSION

Acceptance of our emotions does not mean that we have no choice except to be at the mercy of our bodies as they react to stimuli which produce uncomfortable or painful emotions. On the contrary, once we allow ourselves our feelings, we can choose from a variety of ways to communicate them to others. The most common methods are stating feelings, making sounds, taking appropriate actions, and touching.

Unfortunately, when our brains give our bodies the reactions that accompany anger, fear, or pain, there's little we can do to stop the process. The best, time-proven way to deal with emotions is to express them.

Although it's a tremendous relief to be able to yell or shout when we're fiercely angry, we cannot always find the right time and place to do this. Sometimes simply stating "That makes me angry" or "I don't like it when you do (say) that" provides all the release necessary to achieve serenity.

If you feel timid about taking charge or being assertive, consider this: statistics show that happy, well-adjusted mothers have more contented babies than overly anxious women. With this thought as your motivation, you may find the courage to assert yourself and use your imagination to seek appropriate ways of flushing out the potential poisons of unexpressed emotions.

When sad or fearful, and alone, go to a private place;

groaning, or sobbing, or crying provides a wonderful safety valve. However, it also remains important to communicate these feelings by telling your mate or a close friend about the painful or frightened feelings you have been experiencing.

Finally, remember that pleasure and love need equal time with anger, fear, and pain. A thoughtful card, words of praise, or a special favor will not only make someone else feel better but will also heighten your own positive feelings.

If you have been repressing affection or friendship, make a conscious effort to touch your loved ones. You may want to reserve your kisses and intimate caresses for your mate, but a hand clasp or a hug often expresses more than words can ever say. They give you pleasure as well. Bonding is not the exclusive right of infants. Dr. Casriel comments that every adult has a survival-based need to trust and be connected to others.

Practicing Step 3

Step 3, understanding your emotions, involves the following:

- Developing healthy emotional attitudes
- Identifying emotions
- Expressing emotions

Changing old attitudes is not an easy task. The first time you attempt to sound out anger or pain, you may experience self-consciousness, embarrassment, or even guilt. It's as if a tiny tape recorder in your head constantly tells you to be quiet and behave properly. Turn off the noise. Instead, make emotional sounds and convince yourself, "I'm entitled to have and express all my feelings."

When you loudly utter "Ahhhhhh" or "Ohhhhhh," notice the changes in your breathing. Did your eyes begin to tear? Is your heart beating faster? If so, you probably are experiencing fear, pain, or both. A noisy and strong sound, accompanied by a powerful feeling in your arms and other muscles, usually indicates anger.

If you remain unclear about your feelings, your dreams can provide the answers. For example, the night after our discussion of her problems, Pamela the reporter had this dream:

> Went to my office late at night and to my surprise, my mother was in there, reading the manuscript in my type-writer. She said, "You can't print this! It's terrible! I'll never be able to face my friends if you print this!" I got mad and told her she had no right to be snooping around there, and I didn't care what her friends might say. She started to cry and I just turned my back on her. Then she threw the pages at me. When I bent down to pick them up, there were two little kittens under the papers. One was pink, one was blue. Mom said, "Don't touch them. You're allergic to cats!" (And I woke up.)

Pamela's dreams quite clearly demonstrated a new aware-ness of her emotions. She told me, "The manuscript Mom was reading in the dream was my article about your work. This dream really emphasized for me the way my parents trained me not to show my feelings. And I felt pretty proud of myself for getting angry and standing up for myself in the dream."

Pamela also seemed to be pleased about the fetal symbols of the kittens. "They were so cute!" she told me. "That's the first time I've dreamed about nice little animals since I got pregnant. Guess this means I'm feeling better about it all. And by the way, I'm not allergic to cats." Pamela thought her mother's warning, "don't touch," was her dreaming self's way of recalling just how thoroughly she had been conditioned as a child to inhibit her natural feelings.

After you've practiced expressing your own emotions, reexamine your earlier dream records. You probably will discover fresh interpretations. Particularly note the words you used to describe your dream feelings and try to substitute one of the basic emotions—pleasure and love, anger, fear, or pain—for a vague term. The words "upset, nervous, good, and bad" may become "angry, afraid, and happy or hurt."

Having completed the vitally important step of understanding your emotions, you are now ready to combine all your new dream analysis skills and to explore some of the finer points of dream interpretation.

CHAPTER 6

❖

Step 4: Interpreting Your Dreams

This chapter brings together all the interpretive skills learned so far and adds some finer points of dream evaluation. You'll discover how to use your knowledge of dream symbols, diagramming, and emotions to understand the patterns and levels of dreams as well as the interpretation techniques used by other dream psychologists.

When you complete this step of my program you can consider yourself an "advanced dreamer," one who is in touch with her deeper consciousness.

Patterns in Dreams

My term "patterns" refers to the repetition of a theme in your dreams over a period of time—a week, a month, or longer. If you review your dream diary right now, you probably will notice that your dreams sometimes refer to the same concern or issue experienced during your waking hours. Once you have addressed or resolved this problem or conflict, the themes of your dreams will probably change.

To see how dream patterns emerge, let's look at several

entries from Sonia's dream diary. I have diagrammed one dream according to the directions in Chapter 5. A legal secretary and mother of two children from a previous marriage, Sonia reported this dream in her third month:

At (my office) with (my two kids,) (I) started to take them (home) for a nap. Went out back in the (small parking lot) to get their (bikes) and heard them screaming and crying out by my car. A (small,) green gopherlike (creature) was snapping at them, terrorizing (them.) (I) smashed (it) with a bike tire but (it) didn't die. It just deflated. (I) picked up a green (worm) with yellow dots on its forehead (I) said to it sympathetically, "Oh, (you)re just looking for a (home,) too." And (I) put it down.

At first, Sonia attached little importance to this rather brief dream. "My dreams are usually much longer and have very complicated plots," she explained, "so I thought this one was almost not worth writing down. Besides, the little animal and that worm were so silly." Yet, when I diagrammed the dream by circling all the characters, underlining the action words, and noting the two settings, the dream assumed greater significance.

This emphasizes the fact that all dreams during pregnancy—no matter how short or seemingly absurd—may provide helpful clues to conflicts and problems. Even a very brief dream, like Sonia's, offers all the information you need to discover the source of an anxiety causing you needless stress or tension.

To see how patterns developed in Sonia's dreams, let's

look first at her analysis. Since small animals usually represent the fetus, Sonia guessed that the little creature terrorizing her older children was her unborn child. Sonia's dream actions also show that she was angry with the baby: she smashed the gopher to protect the siblings. Sonia realized she'd been unconsciously worried that her son and daughter from a previous marriage would feel left out or pushed aside by the new baby.

"My husband and I planned this pregnancy," she told me. "But I admit I've been sort of treating the whole thing lightly, around the kids. I don't want them to think all this will keep me from giving them the attention and love they're used to getting. Things have been hard for them as it is, what with my divorce and remarriage, getting settled in with their stepfather, all that." In her dream Sonia brought the gopher-like creature down to size, so to speak, by "deflating" it. She also had been doing this during her waking hours, constantly telling her older children that the new baby would not make much difference in their daily routines.

Afterward, Sonia told me our discussion helped her to realize that she was not allowing either herself or her family to feel the wonderful excitement and anticipation about this pregnancy—out of fear they'd be jealous. The deflated animal aroused Sonia's compassion in the dream. "When I studied this silly dream and the ridiculous little worm," she said, "it suddenly hit me that this small, new life inside me deserves an equal share of our love—a home, too. But even then, I 'put it down,' and I guess I have been putting down this baby, for the kids' sake."

It is also worth noting that Sonia described the setting of this dream as "the parking lot behind my office." At the time, neither of us noticed the significance of the locale. Then, near the end of her second trimester, Sonia reported the following:

> I was on top of a skyscraper in a city. The top was mapped out like they were building some rooms—college dorm-

type rooms—on the top. My roommate was Ruth, the girl who took over my job when I took maternity leave (I'd just started my leave the day before this dream). There were no walls. I looked down on the city below. We were maybe twenty stories up. Ruth was very pleased about going to the edge but I stayed in the center. I wasn't as much afraid as I was cautious.

When we talked about his dream, Sonia commented that being on an unfinished skyscraper seemed to symbolize that she had reached the peak of her pregnancy. "But I'm not ready to even *think* about labor and delivery just yet," she added. "My first two were very difficult births. Maybe that's why, in the dream, I didn't want to look over the edge."

Both of us thought this dream was the first mention of Sonia's career—until we remembered that the earlier dream of the attacking gopherlike creature began at her office. Even then, Sonia had been training Ruth to take over her duties. She told me about her mixed feelings. "Ruth is my friend. I recommended her as a temporary replacement. But sometimes I do think maybe she's, oh, just a little bit *too* good at it. It has occurred to me that she might not want to quit when I'm ready to come back—or that my boss may want her to stay on."

The conflict over career and motherhood is another common source of anxiety many pregnant women experience today. Sonia loved her family, and the prospect of their own child meant a great deal to her new marriage. At the same time, her career was important. "We're going to really need that extra paycheck," she told me. "And I'd care about my job even if we didn't need the money. I started working right after my divorce, and this job gave me the first self-confidence I ever really felt about myself."

By simply examining two dreams from one woman's journal, we can see a pattern that suggests several areas of concern. First, Sonia was worried about the effect of the new baby on her other children; second, she dreaded the possible pain and difficulty of the approaching delivery; additionally, she wanted to continue her career and still be an adequate parent.

Once she understood her sources of anxiety, Sonia took action toward their resolution. She began by talking with other women about the ways they coped with sibling rivalry. In her Lamaze class she discussed the approaching delivery and was reassured that now she would have better care. "This time," she told me, "my husband will be with me during labor. That in itself will make a tremendous difference."

Scrutinize your own dream records for patterns or repetitive themes. If any symbols or themes are repeated, your inner self may be trying to focus your attention on a particular anxiety or problem previously avoided. Do any characters or objects keep popping up? Is the same setting or a similar one mentioned in two or more of your dreams?

Remember that while the symbols may vary, the category or group might be the same. In Sonia's early dream, the gopherlike creature and the little worm were different; still, they both belong in the general category of small animals symbolizing the fetus.

As your pregnancy progresses, your dreams may seem quite different from the earlier ones. For example, the size and appearance of architectural references often change with each trimester.

Buildings and related symbols usually reflect a perception of the body's inner space, especially the enlarging uterus. First trimester dreams may fail to reveal any architecture, since the settings will often be in small, enclosed spaces. When the dream takes place out of doors you may dream you are in a car, bus, boat, or plane—again, a fairly enclosed space.

Sonia's early dream took place in the parking space behind her office. Her second trimester dream found her on top of a skyscraper—a dramatically larger architectural reference corresponding to a rapidly enlarging uterus. Now, notice how the following seventh-month dream continued to reflect the office theme:

> I worked in a government office. It was a very important job. I had my own office, and it was very bright and happy. We were having a meeting in my office, a very relaxed meeting. I think we were even throwing paper cups in the air. There was a lion on a stretcher, unconscious. My Dad walked in because he had some official business with this office. He was very surprised that I was in charge. I didn't even introduce him to my staff or co-workers. Just took care of his business very matter-of-factly and then I left to do some other things. Dad was very dumbfounded! I felt very satisfied.

Recurring themes of this sort usually indicate that the dreamer still cannot find a solution to an ongoing conflict or problem. If you continue to envision similar plots or action—and especially if you're having the same dream—work in earnest to resolve the underlying issues. Once you do this, recurring dreams and themes probably will subside.

When we talked about her government office dream, Sonia explained that her father had never given her the support or approval she felt she deserved. "In this dream I was very casual about Dad's arrival and treated him just as I did any other business guest. In real life, I'm usually desperate for his approval," she commented. "So the dream really helped me see that I can feel good about myself without Dad's acknowledgment. I've outgrown the need for his acceptance. I can support myself and can get the respect and love I need from others."

Having come to terms with family issues, Sonia nevertheless thought the unconscious lion in the government office dream symbolized some unresolved feelings about her pregnancy: "I think the unconscious lion represents my baby, just lying there for the time being. But when that lion wakes up, when that baby is born, watch out! The whole office scene could become chaos!'' Apparently, Sonia was still worried about being able to resume her career when this third child arrived; her dreams continued to remind her of the need to make a decision.

Following is one of the last dreams Sonia recorded before her delivery. Notice the repetition of an office setting and Sonia's ultimate determination to combine motherhood and career.

> At my old office, Ruth (the friend who replaced me at work) was having a few minor problems and my help was enlisted to solve them. Dr. Doe, my obstetrician, had moved his office into half of my old office. I was really delighted I could be there so often, working at both places. While working, we were admiring a yellow Corvette in the parking lot outside. It had a telephone. This phone had a cord or cable that was hooked up to our office. Ruth had to answer it. There was a slightly slanted balcony. I was lying on it and the ocean came up. We were up high but the water was right there.

By now, you probably recognize the numerous symbols related to pregnancy in this example. Some are quite obvious, such as the obstetrician and the ocean, representing labor and the waters breaking, respectively. Also, notice the car, symbolizing Sonia's body, connected to the office with an umbilical-like cord. We thought the slanted balcony might have depicted labor, too, because Sonia's Lamaze instructor emphasized the importance of either squatting or being propped in a slanting position to allow gravity to assist the delivery.

All of these symbols tell us that Sonia's job was almost equally important to her as the new baby. Even the obstetrician had his office connected to Sonia's. The constantly recurring business setting helped this expectant mother decide to return to her job after the baby was born. By working part-time, she was able to continue her professional pursuits and care for her larger family. Meanwhile, her husband advanced in his own career, so Sonia no longer felt obliged to work full-time.

Charlotte, another 35-year-old legal secretary, was troubled by the anger she often expressed in her dreams. In her first trimester, she dreamed of being frustrated while waiting in the supermarket checkout line and began throwing bottles and cans at those ahead of her. Yet, Charlotte was horrified at herself. "I'd never even *think* of doing that in real life," she told me.

These angry feelings continued as Charlotte's pregnancy progressed. In a second trimester dream, she got a shotgun and killed nosy neighbors who were prowling around her backyard. "The woman next door is always giving me unwanted advice," she said, "but I usually just listen and then go on about my business. I can't figure out why I'd dream of shooting her!" Charlotte admitted having difficulty in being attentive to her husband and feared she might lose her temper with him "for some silly reason and then be sorry later." At this point, I persuaded Charlotte to join one of my dream study groups for expectant parents.

During her third trimester Charlotte reported this nightmare:

> I am lost in an underground junkyard. It is like a parking garage but is filled with all kinds of broken furniture, garbage, and wrecked cars. I feel really mad at my husband because he dropped me off here and told me it was a shopping mall. It's a maze of tunnels and I can't find my way out. Then I see an exit sign and start to run toward it. But I trip and fall onto a big pile of scrap metal. Wires and nails catch in my clothes and I can't get up. I feel paralyzed. I try to scream for help but I've lost my voice so nothing comes out. Suddenly this huge machine (like those bulldozers they use to crush wrecked cars) starts coming toward me. The man driving it looks like my doctor. I try to wave to him but he doesn't see me, and the

big crushing machine keeps bearing down on me. (Then
I woke up, feeling really scared but also still a little bit mad
at my husband for no real reason.)

You probably recognize many of the pregnancy and childbirth symbols in Charlotte's nightmare: the underground
setting (her body, especially the uterus), the maze of tunnels
(labor), and her doctor (who was "bearing down" on her,
suggesting the approaching delivery date). When asked to
tell us her associations to a junkyard, broken furniture, gar-
bage and wrecked cars, she said, "They're things nobody
wants any more. Like me, these days." It appeared that
Charlotte had a very low opinion of herself because of her
husband's insensitivity since she became pregnant.

She told us that her spouse had refused to come with her
to childbirth preparation classes, although he willingly
drove her there and picked her up afterward. "The night I
had this nightmare," she recalled, "he had car trouble and
never showed up. I was standing out there in the dark for
nearly an hour, after everyone else had left. Finally I walked
to a phone booth and called him. He was at home watching
TV! All the way home on the bus, I was pretty annoyed with
him. Maybe that's why I had this awful dream."

Like many women, Charlotte had not been allowed to
express anger as a child. Another member of our dream
study group pointed out that being entrapped by a pile of
junk might be symbolic of sitting on or holding in a veritable
stockpile of unexpressed emotions, especially anger.

When she understood the possible effects of this inner
emotional turmoil on her health and that of her baby,
Charlotte decided to take action. She not only told her
neighbor she didn't appreciate all the advice but also persuaded her husband to attend the remaining Lamaze classes
with her. Additionally, Charlotte tried my method of rolling
up her car windows and yelling to release tension. Before the
end of her pregnancy, her frightening dreams subsided.

Charlotte's nightmare also reflected another typical pregnancy fear: loss of control over one's body. This fear became evident when she described her inability to move and the laryngitis. Waving to her doctor for help also represented a less blatant fear. By gradually learning to express her needs and feelings by communicating them to others, however, Charlotte found these anxieties diminishing. She then anticipated delivery with pleasure rather than dread.

DIFFERENT TRIMESTERS, DIFFERENT DREAMS

In general, early pregnancy dreams differ from later ones in that most of the symbols or dream elements are smaller. Sonia's initial fetal symbols (the green gopher, the worm) became larger as her pregnancy progressed (the unconscious lion). The settings of her dreams expanded, too: the parking lot seemed inconsequential compared to the tall skyscrapers and impressive government office of her later dreams. Yet Sonia's dream patterns remained much the same. The recurring themes of her conflict over balancing a career and motherhood continued to dominate the plot, even as concerns about a painful delivery and her relationship with her father also begged her attention.

Although some researchers insist that the dreams of each trimester vary greatly, I have not found such strong demarcations. However, we can make some general observations about the differences occurring during each trimester. Architectural references and fetal symbols do get larger toward the end of the second trimester and into the third. More women also dream about actual human babies rather than plants, growing things, or small animals as they near delivery. There are more striking differences in the settings than in any other dream element.

First trimester dreams may take place in closets and small spaces. For example, here's a "fitting room" dream that Agnes recorded in her second month:

I was in a shopping mall, trying on bathing suits. Looking for a red bikini with a gathered bottom to hide my round tummy but nothing looked right. While I was trying these on in the fitting room, a rat came in from behind the curtain. It looked mean and scared me. (I woke up.)

Agnes obviously was becoming more aware of her pregnancy, and even in her dreams she attempted to camouflage her enlarging tummy (a gathered bikini bottom to hide it). An expectant mother who wanted a child and had planned her pregnancy, she nevertheless maintained typically ambiguous feelings about it all. The rat invading her private space symbolizes a secret revulsion at the idea that another being was taking over her body.

Agnes had another dream within the same period. It provides further insights into her feelings about her changing body.

Dreamed I was in the laundry room of our apartment complex, washing baby things. As I sorted the clothes, my diaphragm fell out. I thought, "I won't need THAT any more!" and felt sad. Then I opened the trash bin to throw it away. Then two white bunnies hopped out of the bin, their claws scratching me. While I was fighting them off, more and more bunnies came tumbling out. There were hundreds! They were stampeding like cattle in a Western movie, hopping all over me. I was crying for help but no one could hear me. (Woke up feeling very scared.)

You may recall that I previously mentioned this episode of stampeding bunnies as an example of exceptions to the general meanings of typical pregnancy dream symbols. In this case, Agnes associated rabbits with sex, and would not agree that they might be fetal symbols. "I think of Playboy Bunnies and all the jokes about rabbits making out all the time," she explained.

Note that this dream's setting was also a relatively small, enclosed space (the laundry room). Once again, small animals frightened Agnes. In our discussion it developed that she was worried that having intercourse somehow might harm the baby. Learning about the different levels of dream symbols, however, Agnes later agreed that the stampeding bunnies might possibly have two meanings: one pertaining to sexual activity and the other to the fetus. Understanding these dimensions is another fine point to be considered as you polish your dream interpretation skills.

Levels in Dreams

Almost all the dreams we've reviewed so far have different levels of meaning. In other words, the same symbols or themes may reflect several issues or concerns. Sometimes even a single element has several levels of meaning for the dreamer. Let's reconsider Agnes' short nightmare of being frightened by a rat while trying on bathing suits in a fitting room. We already know this dream revealed two of Agnes' concerns: upset over her appearance and the invasion of her body.

During our discussion, another group member asked Agnes to define "red bikini" as if addressing someone who'd never heard of the words. Agnes replied, "A bikini is two strips of cloth women with slim figures wear to the beach or pool. It's almost like being nude. And the color red is the same color as ripe apples or tomatoes. It's an exciting, sexy color and I always feel good when I wear it." Did anything in her waking life remind her of these associations, of being nude or exciting and sexy? She replied, "Well, I do feel excited and (excuse the expression) 'horny' a lot lately. But I try to keep those feelings to myself. They're not, well, you know—not maternal."

Agnes might not have admitted these feelings if her husband had been in class that session. Sometimes expectant mothers need people other than their partners when they first begin to express their innermost feelings. Look for a hospital-sponsored pregnancy support group or speak privately to your childbirth preparation instructor. Once you've confided in an understanding person, you will be more inclined to discuss your feelings with your partner; he often shares the same worries.

After being reassured by the other students that her sexy feelings were normal and appropriate for mothers-to-be, Agnes could hardly wait to go home and try them out! One student even pointed out that the dream setting of a fitting room may even have symbolized that nudity and excitement "fit" her now.

At the next class, Agnes' husband Rudy grinned as he told us, "I thought this dream stuff was a waste of time until Agnes told me about what happened here last week. We didn't know about how pregnancy usually makes women feel turned on. It makes sense, though. All that increase in hormones, plus the pressure on her insides." Rudy began to blush. "Anyhow, now I'm all for understanding our dreams and sharing them."

Jackie, the 35-year-old journalist and mother of twins from a previous marriage, had a number of dreams containing several levels. In her fourth month, she reported this one:

My husband David and I were walking along a familiar street. It was in my home territory. Being hungry, we stopped in front of a restaurant. David went in to check it out. If it was okay, he would call me inside. I waited and waited. He didn't come, so finally I went in, anyhow. There was an enormous room inside, with a huge round table in the center that was almost filled with people I knew from my high school days. I was thrilled to see them all. I joined them and we were all talking excitedly when David came over. He had been in the back at the bar and he was reeling drunk. When he introduced himself to my friends it was so embarrassing because he was almost incoherent and stumbling around. Then he excused himself and walked away. I told my friends, "He's not usually like this," and they said, "Well, we should hope not!" I couldn't believe it! The fact is, David never drinks and he's never like that. At that point, I began to think it was all very strange and I felt confused. I didn't know whether I should follow David and see if he needed my help, or if I should enjoy my independence and stay there having fun with my old friends. (The dream sort of faded and I woke up.)

Asked to describe "home territory," Jackie explained that she felt it was not limited only to the town where she grew up. The dream setting seemed to have other dimensions, representing her life from kindergarten through high school.

Describing a restaurant, Jackie said, "It's a place where you're served and nourished." This reminded her of her relationship with David. "Our marriage makes me feel served and nourished. Also—oh, yes! It's our unborn child, because I'm serving and nourishing it in my body."

Jackie went on to define the restaurant table by saying, "It's a large disk supported by wooden sticks for legs, with a cloth on top." Then she stopped and laughed. "That's also just the way one of my twins might draw a picture of a pregnant woman—a large disk with little sticks for legs!"

Jackie had trouble understanding the meaning of David's drunkenness in her dream, until he mentioned that they'd both been attending groups for Adult Children of Alcoholics. Jackie was subconsciously confronting her feelings about her father, who died of alcoholism. "That's it!" she exclaimed again. "Of course. In the dream, David symbolizes my father. My dad was always hanging out in bars. And, David is the only 'father figure' in my life right now. Also, I used to feel the same way when I was a child— confused, and wanting to do my own thing and not being drawn into Dad's needs and problems. And, just as in my dream, I used to feel embarrassed about Dad, the same way I did in the dream when David met my friends."

It's quite evident that a number of concerns surfaced in Jackie's dream: the transition she has made from her former life-style to the present one; the new demands both this second marriage and second pregnancy impose on her role as wife, mother, and nurturer; and the growing awareness that, unlike her father, David is a man she can depend on and trust.

When Jackie discussed her dream of meeting many former friends in a restaurant situated in her "home territory," her first association was of her marital relationship, which served and nurtured her emotionally. At another level, she thought the restaurant symbolized her pregnancy and nourishment of the child within.

The entire setting also represented more than Jackie's hometown. She told us it symbolized "the place and the time when I got all my early training. More than school, it stood for all the people who influenced the development of my personality and was the place where I learned how to relate to others." Jackie went on, "Nowadays I'm learning new ways. Such as that all men aren't like my Dad. And much, much more. I'm a lot different now than I was back there." Jackie thought her dream mainly aimed to dispel the fears she'd experienced in her first pregnancy, because her husband now supports her and she, herself, is a more capable person.

The following excerpts from other pregnant women's dreams demonstrate the concept of levels, or more than one possible meaning for a single dream element:

Stacey, 28-year-old insurance agent, in her third month: There were all kinds of house plants and vases of flowers, dozens of them, flying around in my office, with dirt and water falling all over my important papers . . . worried that the plants and flowers would die.

Krystal, 30-year-old junior high teacher, in her third month: Found a big pile of apples on my desk, making (me) angry . . . the kids were trying to bribe me for better grades. . . . The students were all little toddlers in diapers . . . worms crawled out of the fruit.

Marlise, 27-year-old hospice nurse, in her sixth month: A patient who looked like my mother . . . died with her head on my chest . . . turned into a baby . . . began sucking my breast and it felt wonderful . . . slapped her . . . became Mom again, and cursed at me.

Rosita, 30-year-old homemaker, mother of two, in her eighth month: In a very big restaurant kitchen, dicing tomatoes and peppers for salsa . . . changed into babies' heads and little legs, so cute . . . flushed them down the toilet . . . made (me and husband) sad . . . we cried and cried . . . tried to make more and they changed to babies, too . . . was upset because all of a sudden, I couldn't cook right any more.

Sometimes the various levels of dream elements are quite obvious, as in Stacey's dream of the flying plants (fetal symbols). At one level, she was worried that they would die; at another level, she showed concern about being able to balance a career and motherhood. The conflict was represented by the way the dirt and water, pregnancy symbols, threatened to ruin her important business papers.

One symbol often projects two or more of the dreamer's fears. Marlise, for example, had difficulty sorting out her dying patient's changing faces. Later she saw that this person reflected both her desire to nourish the child (breastfeeding) and her ambiguous feelings about her pregnancy (slapping the baby).

The patient also resembled Marlise's mother, whose health had been failing. After interpreting this dream, Marlise realized she was both sad and angry about her mother's illness. "I'm afraid she won't live to see her first grandchild," Marlise explained, "and I'm also mad that she didn't take better care of herself." Simply sharing these feelings with our group helped Marlise release the anxiety she was experiencing. Afterward, these themes did not recur in her dreams.

When Rosita described her salsa babies, she thought the tomatoes and peppers symbolized the fetus. Then she explained, "Once, I had an abortion and we both felt guilty about it, so that was the salsa going down the toilet, and our sadness. But now we have a new baby coming." As we discussed her dream, Rosita also realized that her inability to cook right—with the vegetables continually becoming inedible—symbolized her fear of being unable to mother three small children. Acting on this realization, Rosita enlisted the help of her younger sister, who agreed to live with the growing family until all the children were out of diapers.

THE IMPORTANCE OF DREAM WORK

If you work or already have other children, you may feel that you don't have time for dream analysis. A working mom in her second pregnancy, Megan was busy with her efforts to run a smooth household, arrange for her first child's day care, perform efficiently in her work, and simultaneously entertain her husband's business associates on weekends. She felt she lacked time to work on her dreams until her obstetrician found she was showing high blood pressure from stress. He began to insist that Megan take early maternity leave.

During this stressful period, she reported this dream:

> I was in a very weird house. (It was ours in the dream but I've never actually seen such a house in real life.) It had dozens of rooms, long hallways, many stories. The floors were tilted, slippery, and hard to walk on. I was trying to get the place cleaned up because guests were coming. Went into a huge ballroom and turned on the vacuum. It made a roaring noise and took off, sucking up rugs and drapes and everything it came across. Looking for the socket to unplug it, saw some mice crawling out of the walls. After I got the vacuum turned off and started hitting the mice with a broom, there was a loud noise in the halls, so I went to see. There was some kind of earthquake, and big oil paintings were crashing down off the walls. The floor split open and I fell down into the basement. (Woke up in a panic. Then, when I managed to get back to sleep, the dream began again! This never happened to me before.) Now I was where I had fallen, in a dark base-

ment. Lit a candle and there were some horrible, indescribable monsters or maybe burglars in the corner, coming after me. (Then I woke up again and was afraid to go back to sleep for the rest of the night.)

This nightmare clearly highlights the stress Megan was feeling as a result of her work overload. As she described her associations, she began to realize how complicated her lifestyle had become. "No wonder my dream house seems weird," she told us. "That's the way I've been feeling about this pregnancy—as if I'm a stranger in my own body. And lots of times I feel as if everything is getting out of control, like the vacuum cleaner."

Megan admitted to typically ambiguous feelings about her pregnancy. "I want this baby so much," she told the class, "but I didn't know I'd have to change my routines to have it." She thought her dream pointed this out by depicting the fetal symbols (mice) in the wall. "It's as if I've tried to tuck the baby out of sight," she commented, "but while I'm rushing around doing all these other really unimportant things, the baby is demanding my attention." Megan believed the earthquake, her fall into the basement, and the threatening intruders all represented the harm that might befall her and her unborn child unless she somehow got relief from stress.

Instead of taking early maternity leave, Megan eliminated the entertaining and persuaded her husband to take over some of the evening and weekend child care. She also began to interpret her dreams as a way to target the sources of stress in her life. After one week of dream work, Megan's blood pressure was normal and her doctor agreed that she could continue working.

If you and your partner are "too busy" to keep your dream diary, analyze your subconscious visions, and practice daily relaxation, now may be the ideal time to slow down. Otherwise, your physical and emotional health could suffer; you may be forced to slow down and pay attention to these issues anyway. Discuss both your schedules and construct a routine that gives you time for these activities. Moreover, sharing your dreams, thoughts, and feelings is excellent insurance for a harmonious relationship.

If you're still having trouble recognizing and interpreting the important elements in your dreams, talk with other expectant moms. When we describe our dreams to someone else, we often suddenly begin to see what they mean. Another person's comments also may shed light on your dream or guide you to new associations. Some famous interpretators base their techniques on these two aspects of dream sharing.

A Look at Other Interpretation Methods

Dr. Montague Ullman, co-author of *Working with Dreams*, uses other people's styles of thinking as the basis for his interpretation method. After one of Ullman's group members describes a dream, peers tell him or her, "If *I* had that dream, it would mean . . ." The dreamer remains silent until everyone else shares personal associations. Then, he or she has the choice of accepting or discarding any of these interpretations. Hearing another person's ideas frequently gives the dreamer a new perspective.

When we tried Ullman's process in my class, Gloria, a 22-year-old homemaker, shared the following:

> I dreamed I was walking along a narrow path through a "tunnel" of trees. The branches of the trees met overhead and formed a kind of ceiling. As I went along, the leaves grew thicker and shut out the sunlight. I began to feel scared because it was getting dark and I kept stumbling. Sharp twigs and branches scratched me and I started worrying that something might happen to the baby. I began running, trying to get out, looking for the end of the tunnel. I could see a little bit of light at the end, but it seemed too far. I was afraid the trees would hurt me before I could reach the end. (I woke up still frightened.)

Before Gloria told us her own interpretation, each of the other students commented, pretending that they themselves had had the dream. Carmen, a student in her first trimester, said, "The long, long tunnel would stand for the way I feel about my pregnancy. It seems a very long time before I'll ever get to the end!" Most of the other women gave similar interpretations.

Then Gloria's husband Martin told us, "If I had that dream, I'd associate the narrow pathway and the scary tunnel with Gloria's labor. Our doctor told us her pelvis may be too small and she may have to have a C-section. So I've been worried about that and how I'll be able to handle it if it happens. The scratching twigs and three limbs make me think of the ordeal that's coming soon, since Gloria is due in three weeks. The tunnel might represent the birth canal and the difficulty the baby may have trying to come out through a narrow passage."

When she heard her husband's remarks, Gloria's eyes filled with tears. "That's exactly how I feel," she told us. "But I didn't know Martin felt the same way or that he knows how worried I've been." (As it happened, the couple's six pound, three ounce baby girl was born vaginally, after a reasonably brief labor of 12 hours.) By sharing their dreams, Gloria and Martin also expressed their hidden fears. Gloria told us she hadn't admitted the nightmare's meaning to herself until Martin voiced it first.

Audrey was another group member who joined us in practicing the Ullman technique. A 33-year-old bank teller in her eighth month, Audrey related this dream:

> I am pedaling, going up a steep hill in an adult-sized car which is like a kiddie car. (I am pregnant in the dream.) Trying to reach a well at the top of the hill and it is very difficult because of my weight. The sun is hot; I am so thirsty. It seems to take forever to get there. Along the way I pick a beautiful rosebud, but after it's in the car, it turns out to be a watermelon which I cannot open. Finally I get to the top and the well. Reaching for the bucket, I

fall down the well into cool water. Can't swim, begin to
choke (and then I woke up in a panic).

According to Ullman's method, the other group members
presented their ideas before Audrey gave her own analysis.
Gloria said, "If I had that dream, the struggle up the hill
would symbolize getting to the end of my pregnancy. And
I guess falling down the well, not being able to swim, and
choking would be my fears about the delivery."

In her eighth month also, Claudia suggested, "The car
would remind me of my body, which is getting to be very
hard to manipulate, just like a kiddie car. And I think the
rosebud is a symbol of an adorable little baby."

Then Carmen added, "Yes, and notice how the rosebud
turned into a big ole watermelon, just like our bellies do! But
I don't know what the bucket means, or the hot sun, because
the weather right now is cold and rainy."

When Audrey gave us her analysis, she said, "Almost
everything everybody said gave me good ideas. I also think
the struggle up the hill is about my pregnancy, because I'm
feeling so impatient for it to be over now that it's just one
month away. By the way, in another month it probably will
be really hot weather! And, I agree the rosebud is the baby.
And the watermelon, too. That's also my womb, so big
now—and so is the bucket at the well. But I didn't think I
was worried about labor. What Gloria said has got me wondering."

As our discussion turned to fears of labor and delivery
pains, Audrey blurted out, "Two things that really worry me
sick are the waters breaking and that I might have to have
an episiotomy. Ugh! The idea of that, just even thinking
about it, makes me feel faint!"

Claudia, who already had had one child, spoke up. "The
waters breaking doesn't hurt at all," she explained. "In fact,
it feels good even though it can be rather messy. It's sort of
like a rubber band bursting. A lot of pressure and tension
just go away with a pop, and it's over. Quite a relief!"

Jeremy P. Tarcher, Inc.
Audio Renaissance Tapes, Inc.
9110 Sunset Boulevard
Los Angeles, California 90069

If you would like to learn more about
Jeremy P. Tarcher and Audio Renaissance Tapes,
simply complete and mail this card to us.
We will be happy to send you a catalog.

PLEASE PRINT

NAME _____

ADDRESS _____

CITY & STATE _____

ZIP _____

In which title did you find this card?

BOOK _____

TAPE _____

She continued her reassurances by adding, "My Lamaze instructor says not everyone needs an episiotomy. It's only done to widen the birth canal, to keep you from tearing if the baby's head is too large or if the baby is coming very fast, and the doctor gave me a local painkiller first." When she saw Audrey's horrified expression, Claudia went on, "You won't feel that injection at all, I promise you, because you'll be so dilated, so stretched, you'll be numb there anyway, believe me."

Claudia's reassurances were accurate for the most part. Her description of the bag of waters breaking fits the general impression most mothers report. However, the episiotomy procedure has recently been a topic of controversy among obstetrical caregivers. Carl Jones, Bradley childbirth educator, and author of *Mind Over Labor,* frowns upon physicians who routinely make these incisions. Instead, Jones suggests massaging the perineum area during pregnancy and avoiding taking a supine position (with feet in stirrups) during labor. Lamaze teachers also emphasize the importance of allowing gravity to do much of the work—by sitting up, squatting, or using a birthing chair—especially during the last stages of labor.

Although her own Lamaze instructor had described both the waters breaking and episiotomy, Audrey had been too shy to voice her fears in class. She told us that our frank group discussions made it easier for her to admit these worries. As it turned out, Audrey gave birth to a healthy, six-pound baby boy, without the need for an episiotomy. During our postpartum interview, she told me, "I can't believe I worried about the waters breaking. It was just like Claudia said, a real relief when it happened. Ever since that dream study group, I've learned to speak up and ask questions now if anything worries me, even if it makes me blush a little."

In another very effective method devised by Gayle Delaney, Ph.D., author of *Living Your Dreams,* group members ask one participant to choose a dream element (a setting or character) and describe it as if the group were aliens from outer space. This technique helps the dreamer focus on many issues that might not have occurred to her otherwise.

When we tried the Delaney method in one of my groups, Vanessa, a 20-year-old waitress in her sixth month, told us this dream:

> I was going to the city on a ferry, on the top deck. The bay was very choppy and I felt seasick, so I went below. Sat and put my head between my legs. A man next to me asked if he could help. I looked up and saw Tom Selleck, right there beside me! I was thrilled, to put it mildly. He gave me a cup of cool water and asked when the baby was due. I lied, "I am not pregnant, not really. This is just a costume for a play I'm going to be in today in San Francisco." Then he asked all these questions about the play. Of course I couldn't answer. I was embarrassed and started to cry (and woke up.)

When describing Tom Selleck to us as if we were aliens from Mars, Vanessa said, "He's a very handsome man, a movie actor, very sexy, very nice. I just saw him in *Three Men and a Baby.*" Did he remind her of anyone in her waking life? "Actually, I know several people who look a little like him," she responded. "My husband Henry, and also Tim, the man I went steady with before I married Henry. Also, my obstetrician looks kind of like Tom Selleck." When pressed for more details, Vanessa said, "Oh, of course! Both Tim and Henry didn't want me to get pregnant. I had a miscarriage when I was living with Tim, in my third month, and we broke up after that, mainly because he never wanted kids. Then, Henry wanted to wait until he's making more money, so when I found out I'm pregnant, I didn't tell him at first. So the dream must be about that. About the way I tried to hide it from him at first, the way I tried to convince Tom Selleck in the dream that I was wearing a pregnant-looking costume."

As we continued to interview Vanessa, she readily identified other symbols and themes. She thought the boat referred to her pregnancy, with the choppy bay waters symbolizing the labor to come. At another level, her pretense of not being pregnant reflected the ambivalence about parenthood so typical of many expectant mothers. "I want this baby, I really do," she explained, "but I worry that Henry might feel overloaded with the expense. He already had to quit going to night school for his B.A. so he could work an extra shift. So sometimes I do wish I hadn't gotten pregnant so soon."

Vanessa also realized that her dream predicament—pretending to be in a play she knew nothing about—had a definite resemblance to her views on becoming a mother. "I feel like I'm playing a part, only I don't know the script," she told us. "Until I got to Lamaze class and this dream group, I didn't know any other pregnant women. The other waitresses where I work are all teenagers and none of them have ever been pregnant. And, I just never took care of little babies so I don't know if I can handle it."

Fear of being an inadequate parent is another major source of anxiety to many pregnant women. Like Vanessa, they often suffer needlessly until they attend a childbirth preparation class in the last trimester. They finally learn that such concerns remain common and that there are numerous free or inexpensive ways to prepare themselves for the care of a tiny newborn.

Another expectant mother secretly troubled by a typical pregnancy anxiety, Eve feared losing her mate. A nightmare depicted her in an open field with her husband, sister, and hundreds of other people. Suddenly, nearly everyone died, except for Eve, her sister, and a few others. Those who lived were weeping, mourning. Then a miracle happened:

> Out of the ground a goddess rose up. She could see our suffering, so she gave us back our loved ones for one day. We danced and sang and made love. Then all who had died started walking up the hill. I ran up and saw Donald (my husband) standing behind this barrier. I tried to jump

over it but couldn't because it was too high and because of the baby. I searched for the goddess. I yelled out, "Why me? Why always me?" A ray of sunshine hit the ground and the goddess rose up, encased by dirt. You could see her white gown underneath. She said, "You may kiss me, but do not touch me." So I kissed her cheek, then she floated away. (When I woke up, I had to wake my husband just to be sure he was really alive. This was an awful nightmare—had a hard time going back to sleep.)

Using the Delaney method, Eve described her dream goddess: "She is ethereal, almost angelic, just as I imagine my Dream Power. This is the way I visualize the part of myself that gives me dreams: a tall, beautiful woman in a silky white Grecian-style gown." When asked if the goddess reminded her of anyone in her waking life, Eve said, "Oh! I just remembered! I had a dress almost like that when Donald and I were first dating. He even told me I 'looked like a goddess' in that dress."

Thus it occurred to Eve that the heavenly power might be her. Furthermore, she revealed a fear of losing her husband, whose father had died of a sudden heart attack. Her own beloved father had died when Eve was a child. At another level, Eve thought that this dream symbolized her ability to hold her husband's love, despite fears that he might leave her. She reached a comforting conclusion as she related the nightmare: although she lost her husband in the dream, by appealing to her better self, the goddess, she was able to have him returned.

Even women who are self-sufficient before pregnancy find themselves becoming increasingly dependent on the expectant father. "I had to stop working sooner than I'd planned," Eve told me. "Now I depend on my husband for all kinds of small things. It's not just the money he makes to support us, it's things around the house that I used to do myself. It makes me feel so, well, so *vulnerable.* I can't help thinking, what if something happened to him? How on earth would I manage?"

Eve's nightmare also reflected emotional pain, with all the female characters grieving for their loved ones. She thought this also might symbolize her typically ambivalent feelings about starting a family. "We really want this baby," she explained, "but we both sometimes wish we could go out and party all night the way we did when we were first married." She sighed, "Maybe I'm grieving for the freedom we once had. Guess those days are gone forever!"

However, after Eve and Donald's healthy baby girl was born, she told me her mother and sister volunteered to baby-sit, allowing the couple to resume their social life. "But now," she said, "we don't even want to party as much as we used to. We're closer than ever, having gone through the delivery together. And we both just love being a real family and staying at home together."

Practicing Step 4

The fourth step in our understanding of dreams and other states of consciousness during pregnancy brings together all the techniques mentioned in previous chapters. Additionally, it is important to notice the emergence of dream patterns by looking at your diary over a period of several weeks or longer.

As your pregnancy progresses, you will probably notice recurring themes, sometimes disguised beyond easy recognition. Look for similar settings, with particular attention to architectural references, similar emotions (especially in relation to fetal, pregnancy, and childbirth symbols), and similar characters.

Next, notice the different "levels" of concerns in your dreams. The same element may have several associations for you, all of which seem to ring true. The presence of a particular object or character could represent dual meanings, just as Agnes' red bikini symbolized both a worry about her appearance and her enhanced sexual feelings.

If you're still having difficulty discovering the hidden

meaning of your dreams, talk them over with your partner and others. Some couples find that these discussions can be an absorbing and entertaining way to spend an evening. It's also fun to try out a variety of group techniques, such as the methods developed by Ullman and Delaney. Along the way, you probably will enjoy discovering more about other people's innermost feelings, fears, hopes, and creativity. Most important, however, you will gain a deeper understanding of your own dreams and the wise messages your inner self is sending you.

CHAPTER 7

❖

Step 5: Working with Your Dreams

Using your dreams to help you pinpoint the sources of unexpressed anxiety is not the only benefit of my five-step program. Once you've mastered the interpretation skills of the first four steps, you can learn to actually control your dreams in order to

- Discover the meaning or purpose of any dream element
- Dream about a subject of your choice
- Program yourself to have a healing dream
- Request specific information from your dreaming self
- Direct the action, setting, and characters of your dreams

Step 5 of my program consists of learning to employ the dream-incubation and lucid-dreaming techniques. The incubation of a dream (an especially appropriate term for pregnant women) involves focusing on the topic of your choice. A lucid dream is one in which you realize you are dreaming during the dream. In addition to practicing these amazing, yet remarkably easy, techniques, you will learn how to foster your personal "dream power," that wise and imaginative part of your inner self responsible for creating visions.

Dream Incubation

Incubation simply means that an individual decides on a desired dream topic, falls asleep, and then captures the vision. Basically, this technique consists of telling yourself, just as you're drifting off, what you wish to dream about.

Dream researchers theorize that the brain's right hemisphere is more accessible and open to suggestion when our bodies are deeply relaxed. As explained in Chapter 2, this part of the mind helps assign various meanings to the images and signals received from the brain stem when we sleep. If given a direct suggestion about a dream topic, the right brain usually obliges. When this occurs, we have successfully incubated a dream.

Dream incubation dates to the ancient Greeks, who made pilgrimages to temples of Aescalepius, the god of healing. After various rituals designed to cleanse their bodies and minds, the visitors then slept in a sacred room where they were supposed to have a healing dream or receive instructions for recuperating.

There's no need for you to make a pilgrimage to a Greek temple, however, to incubate a dream. Psychologist Patricia Garfield says that a belief in its accomplishment is more important than any other ritual. I also would add another requirement: deep relaxation. My adaptation of Dr. Garfield's and other psychologists' methods is especially effective with pregnant women, who are already more in touch with right-brain powers than most other people.

One of my students who successfully incubated dreams was Julianna, a 27-year-old advertising copywriter in her second pregnancy. During her third trimester she recorded this nightmare. Julianna had just attended her weekly Lamaze class:

It was Saturday and I wasn't working. Mom came to visit so we put Junior in his playpen on the patio and started to have lunch out there. Then a little lizard slid out and crawled to the playpen. I got up to kick it away. Suddenly it began to grow. I backed away, horrified. It got as big as a dinosaur and looked like one, only it was dripping with slimy greenish stuff. Mom started screaming. The monster roared, swished its tail, and spattered her and Junior with that slimy stuff. The baby started crying. (I woke up, just scared out of my wits, and had to get up and see if the baby was all right. The new baby inside me was jumping around as if it might be scared, too.)

Earlier the night of her dream, Julianna's Lamaze instructor had displayed pictures of the fetus in the first stages of growth. Julianna undoubtedly realized that the monster lizard of her nightmare symbolized the fetus. (Interestingly, four other women in class also submitted dreams about reptilian creatures on the same night. This was unusual: no other studies of pregnant women have reported such a strong coincidence in the similarity of dream symbols.) Julianna told me one of the students had commented that the fetus in its early stages looked like a lizard or amphibian. "But why did it attack us like that?" she wondered.

To find out, the next night Julianna incubated a dream about the lizard, with this result:

Once again I was on the patio with Mom and my baby son. This time my husband was there too. And we had a large swimming pool (wish we actually had one, in real life). Then the huge lizard rose up in the middle of the pool. It had large, brown eyes just like Junior's. This time, it was very still and quiet. I wasn't afraid this time, either. I got into the pool and swam over to it. While I treaded water, I asked it, "Why did you frighten us yesterday?" It blinked its big eyes and said in a squeaky, babyish voice, "I need you, too." I felt annoyed and told it, "That's just like a child, you know, having a tantrum to get attention." (And I woke up feeling like laughing about the whole thing.)

This incubated dream helped Julianna confront her fears that the second child would diminish her love for the first, and that she might not be able to care for them both. Once she identified her conflict about the pregnancy, Julianna resolved it by enrolling her first child in a local hospital's program for siblings. She also located other expectant parents who were facing the same possible dilemma. Together, these parents formed a support group with guidance from the hospital staff's counselors and pediatricians.

Even if you believe you do not have any unresolved problems or unexpressed anxiety, it's very rewarding—and a lot of fun—to incubate dreams. Many of my students say they have "met" their unborn babies this way, giving their relationship an advanced start on developing deep love and emotional bonding.

INCUBATION INSTRUCTIONS

Before retiring, make your usual entries in your dream diary: (1) a brief summary of the day's negative thoughts; (2) reversal of these into positive statements; and (3) creation of a positive daydream.

Now, write a description of the topic you wish to feature in tonight's fantasy. Like Julianna, you may want to find out the meaning of a previously troubling dream or you may want to request an explanation for the stress or tension you've been feeling recently for no apparent reason. Perhaps you want to learn more about your baby, your partner, or someone else. Anything you choose can become the subject of your dreams. Once you've selected a topic and written a description, follow these easy steps:

1. First, compose a short, clear sentence describing the intended dream. For example, Julianna wrote, "I will dream about the monster lizard again and I'll

ask it why it frightened my mother and child." Do not ask or plead, merely state your goal. By affirming that you *will* dream about something, you reinforce your mind's determination to provide the information you need. This is one of the reasons it remains so important to believe you can incubate dreams.

2. Having described the dream you want, settle down for sleep. If accustomed to using one of the deep relaxation techniques from Chapter 3, do so now. Otherwise, follow your usual bedtime routine.

3. If your partner knows about the dream incubation experiment, you may wish him to repeat your sentence over and over, very softly, until you have fallen asleep. Just as another person's voice facilitates the integration of a positive daydream, so it can be very effective in directing your mind to create a specific dream. If your partner cannot narrate for any reason, simply repeat the sentence mentally, over and over, until you fall asleep. This repetition boosts your dream-building determination and also encourages drowsiness.

4. When you awaken, try to remain quite still and keep your eyes closed a few moments. Recall what you were just dreaming. Then open your eyes and get up slowly. Write the dream memory in your diary as soon as possible. If you have time, note your associations to it. If not, put the diary aside and come back to it later in the day.

5. *A word of advice:* don't be discouraged if your first attempts are unsuccessful. After trying to incubate a dream, the solution to the problem or conflict may simply pop into your head, even though your initial recall faltered. It may be that once the inner self has been alerted to an issue, it can provide a direct answer without the need for symbolizing it in a dream. Or perhaps you actually experienced

the desired visitor and your waking consciousness has already integrated its message and proposed a solution. Barring these possibilities, you may find the answer to your request in the next dream you remember.

6. Give yourself a mental pat on the back for trying to incubate a dream, no matter what the outcome. Better still, write a sentence or two in your diary, congratulating yourself on undertaking this attempt at dream control.

Self-encouragement cannot be overemphasized. Many Americans still view dreams and their study with suspicion or skepticism, despite the fact that this discipline has been an acceptable scientific endeavor since the 1950s. Since our society does not give us this encouragement, we need to give it to ourselves.

FINDING YOUR PERSONAL DREAM POWER

Once, years ago, when I was facing a block in my own dream work, I decided to practice the suggestions of the well-known dream psychologist Ann Faraday, author of *The Dream Game* and *Dream Power,* by envisioning my own "dream power." Faraday explains that visualizing part of the mind as a separate self or person enables us to contact its thoughts directly.

Closing my eyes, I imagined that my dreaming self was sitting in an empty chair opposite me. My mind initially created a beautiful goddesslike creature with regal bearing, wearing Grecian robes and a benign expression. Since her authoritative, dignified appearance implied a mystical energy, I immediately realized she must be my personal dream power.

I asked her, "Why won't you let me remember my dreams?" Then, still following Faraday's directions, I got up, took the goddess' seat, and pretended to be her. Imagining myself in her lovely diaphanous gown, I shrugged and said, "Why should I help you? You don't have much respect for me! You never place much importance on the dreams I cre- ate, so why should I permit you to recall them?"

Returning to my chair, I humbly asked, "Please, allow me to remember my dreams. In turn, I promise to give them my serious attention." I have had no problems recalling my dreams since that time. Enlisting the aid of this dream god- dess when I incubate dreams, I think of her as a sage and loving friend, standing by with words of wisdom and humor.

If your own efforts to recall or incubate dreams seem futile, try envisioning your own dream power. Your image probably will be completely different from mine, but what- ever the case, the first attempt is usually best.

For example, Agnes' husband Rudy (described in the pre- vious chapter) told us that the person he saw when he tried this technique was a white-haired, bearded, elderly gentle- man who looked like his grandfather. Rudy preferred to call this dream advisor "Papa," the name he had given to his beloved grandfather as a child. After envisioning Papa, Rudy told him, "Tonight I'll dream about my boss. Papa, please help me find a way to ask for more time off so I can be with Agnes for our Lamaze classes." That night, Rudy had this dream.

> Dreamed I was out at the construction site where my company is under government contract to build a new reservoir. There was this enormous, empty excavation and it was my job as engineer to fill it with pure water. I had to do this by carrying buckets of water from a nearby artesian well. I was sweating and straining and getting nowhere. Some hardhats, the workers who did the exca- vation, were sitting on their bulldozers and trucks, off on the side, laughing at me. Then my boss drove up and got out of his car. As he approached me, one of the hardhats yelled to him, "Hey boss, have pity on the poor guy! He needs some help. Whatsa matter with you? It'd be cheaper

to let us lay a pipeline for him." My boss stopped and thought. Then he looked at me and said, "Sounds like a smart idea. What do you think, Rudy?" (Then I woke up, feeling really excited because I could see a way to give a new plan to my boss, a plan that would be cheaper for him and would cut down on my overtime at work.)

Rudy explained that his engineering surveys required his spending long hours either at home or at his office, making computations. He reviewed his time sheets and was able to show his employer that the cost of a new computer system would be less than the overtime fees he was now receiving. "Right now," Rudy told us, "that little bit of extra money didn't seem as important as my being able to go to Lamaze classes—and this class, too—with Agnes. And the best thing was, my boss not only agreed, he also gave me a raise! So it turned out everybody was happy. And all because of the ideas I got from that dream."

In addition to dreaming about your baby or some other person, or about the solution to a problem or conflict, you can learn to use your dreams for healing, as the ancient Greeks did.

HEALING DREAMS

In my work with expectant parents, there have been a few reports of dreams which indicated possible physical complications, even though the dreamers' physicians had not detected any abnormalities. I always urge the individual to schedule an additional check-up when these signs occur.

If you feel embarrassed about describing such a dream to your doctor, simply say that you have been concerned and that another check-up would reassure you. Often, nightmarish dreams of miscarriage, fetal damage, or other frightening symptoms only symbolize another problem or perhaps represent irrational, repressed fears.

For example, Coretta, one of my students, complained of

severe headaches, a condition she had not experienced prior to her pregnancy. Her obstetrician was unable to find any physical cause for the problem. In an effort to get relief, Coretta incubated a dream with this sentence: "I will dream about the cause of my headaches." Following is the result:

> I dreamed I was in a little boat at a lake in the park. It was one of those silly boats that you propel with pedals, like a tricycle. My husband Jerry was in another boat just like mine, right beside me. I told him, "You should pedal harder. I'm getting way ahead of you." Jerry leaned back and grinned at me, in a teasing kind of way. He said, "This is my day off. I just want to relax and enjoy the ride." That made me mad so I pedaled even harder and shot out way ahead of him. Then I looked back and he was nowhere in sight. My legs hurt and my head was splitting and I started to cry. I felt scared and lonely (and I woke up).

When Coretta related this dream, she complained that she was disappointed. "I know it's telling me to relax, or something like that," she said. "But it didn't tell me the cause of these headaches. In fact, this dream gave me a headache! When I woke up my head was throbbing, just like it does every day after lunch."

Another student asked Coretta how she felt after her midday repast, aside from the headaches. The reply was: "Oh, kind of drowsy and heavy, like I could take a nap. But the sleepiness goes away after an hour or so and I'm okay in time to cook dinner or do my other chores." When several women told her they habitually took afternoon siestas, Coretta exclaimed, "Oh, I couldn't do that! I'd never get my work done. Besides, people who do that are lazy. I couldn't lie around like that every day!"

After much persuasion by the other students—and even by Jerry, her husband—Coretta agreed to rest every afternoon, before the onset of her headaches. The next week she told us the problem was gone. "Jerry really doesn't care if everything isn't perfect," she commented. "So I may as well do like he was in my dream—relax and 'enjoy the ride.' After the baby comes, I may not have much time for indulging myself like this."

Lucid Dreaming

A lucid dream is one in which the individual remains almost alertly awake during the dream. Although you may not recall having a lengthy lucid dream, you probably remember occasions when something seemed so extraordinary that you said or thought, "This must be a dream!" Instead of waking up at that point, if you could have continued the fantasy and been aware that you were doing so, you would have experienced a true lucid dream.

Some people possess a natural ability to achieve this state, while others must learn from the directions of dream psychologists. Dr. Jayne Gackenback, a psychology professor at the University of Northern Iowa, conducted experiments indicating that women have more success in lucid dreaming than men.

Dr. Stephen LaBerge, author of *Lucid Dreaming,* first studied his own patterns and those of volunteers in Stanford University's Sleep Laboratory. He then developed a systematic, easy process designed to help anyone have lucid dreams.

DIRECTIONS FOR LUCID DREAMING

While there are several methods now being taught in workshops, the students with whom I've worked favor my adaptation of Dr. LaBerge's MILD (Mnemonic Induction of Lucid Dreams) technique. This method receives attention in the paragraphs that follow. It is important to remember, however, that you first must learn to recall at least four dreams per week and incubate at least two dreams before you'll be ready to have lucid dreams.

1. First, upon awakening, stay in bed with your eyes closed. Mentally review the last dream you can remember. If this happens to be an incubated dream, so much the better. Whatever the results, continue to the next step.
2. Repeat over and over to yourself, with your eyes still closed, "In my next dream, I want to *know* that I am dreaming."
3. Now think of the dream you just recalled and imagine that you are experiencing it again. *Do not ponder how the dream might be different.* Simply recall it in as much detail as possible and imagine that you *know you are dreaming* this time around.
4. Allow yourself to drift back to sleep if you feel drowsy. Merely continue to go over and over your recent dream, imagining that you know you are dreaming. In all likelihood, you'll experience the same episode again. Simply knowing that it is a "rerun" should alert you to the fact that you are dreaming. Then you may wish to change the action or question some of the puzzling characters.

A number of my students who became adept with the MILD technique reported that they encountered lucid dreams totally different from the one they had upon awakening. Although they failed to repeat the first episode, they still knew they were dreaming. With practice, they also developed skill in directing the action and questioning dream characters.

I must offer a word of advice here: as with dream incubation, do not be discouraged if your efforts prove unsuccessful. Only a few of my students or clients have been able to learn to have lucid dreams with any degree of consistency. However, the few women who did learn to induce lucid dreams were able to remain asleep and to actually direct their dream action and characters. These students previously had shown advanced, daily recall powers. They also could incubate dreams about any topic or action they wished. Unless you attain the same level of skills, it's unlikely that you will succeed in creating a lucid dream.

The rewards of lucidity are certainly worth the effort, however. For example, Donna, a 28-year-old restaurant cashier, reported especially vivid and richly detailed dreams. Learning to recall as many as three or more each morning, she had already incubated several dreams that helped her resolve a problem she was having with her mother-in-law.

On this occasion, Donna wanted to dream about her baby. "Every time I try to incubate a baby dream, I get all kinds of little animals and sometimes big ones, too," she complained. "I want to see my real, human baby, the way some of the other women in class have." After several attempts, Donna finally reported this beautiful dream:

(Last night I told myself I wanted to dream about our baby, and I wanted to realize I was dreaming. I said these thoughts over and over to myself until I fell asleep.) Sometime near morning, I dreamed my abdomen became transparent and I could see our baby floating inside. Immediately I knew I was dreaming because this couldn't happen in real life. Then I woke up. I was so disappointed! I told myself over and over I wanted to dream it again, and to stay asleep. Right away I dreamed of the baby in my uterus again, only this time I was there, too. Again, I knew I was dreaming—only this time I didn't wake up. We were floating or swimming underwater, but I could breathe and talk. It was amazing. The water was pale blue and our baby was glowing pink. The cord was sort of a turquoise color, luminescent. It was breathtaking, so beautiful! Then I said to the baby, "Turn over, darling, so I can see if you're a boy or girl." The baby smiled and rolled its little body toward me. It was a boy with long dark hair and huge blue eyes. (Then I woke up with a feeling of reverence and gratitude for this wonderful miracle.)

Yes, Donna's baby did turn out to be a boy, and she said he was born with a lot of long, fine, dark baby hair that turned blond as he got older. If you should be one of those unusual dreamers who succeeds in attaining lucidity, be prepared for an entire new world of sensations, feelings, and insights.

For example, Mila, a 36-year-old loan officer in a bank, was experiencing nightmares about her baby's health. She had undergone amniocentesis and had been told that both she and the baby were fine. Yet she continued to worry that something might go wrong: perhaps the baby would be deformed or she might miscarry. Mila even incubated several dreams, all of which confirmed the baby's health.

Then, in her eighth month, Mila dreamed that she was at a funeral and that a baby was in the coffin. When she awoke that morning, she deliberately remained quiet, eyes closed, to review her nightmare. She repeated silently to herself, "In my next dream, I want to know that I'm dreaming." The following is Mila's lucid dream:

> I am in the same cemetery, but there is no coffin, just a hole in the ground. Some workmen are shoveling dirt into the hole. I ask them, "What happened to the coffin that was here before?" (At that point, I knew I was dreaming. It was the most amazing feeling. I knew because otherwise I wouldn't have remembered about the coffin.) One man says, "That was a mistake. There was no corpse in it." Then I tell him I saw a dead baby in it. He tells me, "You must have been dreaming, lady!" They go back to their shoveling and I notice the hole is now filled with water and floating blossoms. There's a little boy about two years old swimming in the hole. The men pick him up, hand him to me, and say, "This must be what you saw, lady. See? He's alive and well!" The little boy is dripping wet, but I don't mind. I dry him with my shirt and hug him. Then he puts his little arms around my neck and says, "Mommy, I wuv you." (And I woke up, crying with relief

and feeling really happy for the first time in many months.)

Mila believed this dream was telling her (through the workmen) that she had allowed her imagination to make her anxious and depressed. She felt the cemetery hole filled with water, dirt, and flowers (symbols of fertility and growing things) represented her pregnancy. "I think the two-year-old was my baby," Mila told us, "and was that big because I've been worried that I won't be able to take care of a newborn. I have had some experience baby-sitting toddlers. Also, it was really wonderful that he could talk and tell me he loved me."

After this unusual dream, Mila stopped worrying and no longer had nightmares about her baby's health. "It's funny," she said, "that all the medical talk and all my doctor's kind words couldn't make me believe everything is okay. It took this amazing dream to do that." Mila's seven-pound, one-ounce baby boy was born after a nine-hour labor—perfectly healthy.

Finally, a last word of caution about the practical uses of both lucid and incubated dreams. Some pregnant women get very enthusiastic because they assume they can change all their nightmares into happy dreams or destroy the scary monsters by using these techniques. I do not advise pursuing incubation or lucidity for this purpose. Just as happens when we try to repress a strong emotion, an inhibited or destroyed dream element will likely recur in another form.

Even our nightmares have a purpose. Their frightening qualities may be the only way our dreaming self succeeds in capturing our attention. Certainly, we tend to recall weird or scary dreams more readily than we do the happier, calmer variety. Whatever the reason, these symbols or images represent some important factor in our waking lives, some conflict or problem needing our attention.

Rather than incubating dreams in which we attack or destroy these "monsters," it seems a better strategy to befriend them and to attempt to find out the message they want us to receive. For example, in Julianna's incubated dream she made no attempt to hurt the lizard or get rid of it. Instead, she asked it to explain why it had frightened her child and mother. The lizard obliged.

With the completion of this chapter, you have now explored all five steps of my program for understanding your dreams.

Practicing Step 5

Once you have mastered the techniques of dream recall and have begun practicing the finer points of interpretation, you'll be ready to learn to control your dreams. This chapter covered two methods of dream control.

The first, dream incubation, consists of (1) following the nightly routine of writing negative thoughts, changing them into positive ones, creating an affirmative daydream, choosing a topic you wish to dream about, and writing a simple sentence describing your intention; (2) relaxing and repeating the sentence over and over as you drift off to sleep; (3) upon awakening, remaining still for a few minutes, eyes closed, and recalling the dream; (4) arising slowly and writing it in your diary; and (5) being sure to give yourself approval and encouragement for trying to incubate a dream.

If you didn't succeed, try again tonight. Incubated dreams are comparatively easy for most expectant parents. Once you've successfully done it, the ability to exert control over your dreams becomes easier.

The second method of dream control is lucid dreaming. While this technique is more difficult, it can be achieved with perseverance by (1) remaining still upon awakening, with closed eyes, and reviewing the dream you just had; (2) mentally repeating, "In my next dream, I want to *know* I'm dreaming"; (3) again, reviewing the most recent dream and imagining yourself alert to the fact that you're dreaming; and (4) allowing yourself to drift back to sleep.

If you do get a rerun of the episode and become aware you're dreaming, change the action or talk with the dream characters.

In practicing both techniques, you should mentally congratulate yourself for the effort. You are embarking on a difficult journey to learn more about your inner self; the rewards of this journey remain multidimensional. Even if you do not succeed in creating a lucid dream, the attention given to your deeper levels of consciousness can nevertheless help you become more self-confident and loving. These are two important traits every expectant parent should have, both for inner peace and for the relaxation needed for an easier childbirth.

Part Three, "Resolving the Six Fears," will now explain in more detail the thought processes occurring when you're awake and how you can work with them—as well as with your dreams—to alleviate anxiety. These chapters will help you identify the negative waking attitudes so often reflected in your dreams. By changing them, you can relax and enjoy your pregnancy.

PART THREE

❖

Resolving

❖

the

❖

Six

❖

Fears

❖

CHAPTER 8

❖

Coping with the Major Fears of Pregnancy

After studying the first two parts of this book, you may feel you already have resolved some of the major sources of anxiety most pregnant women experience. Some of the expectant mothers I counsel find that, by simply admitting their concerns, fear and stress seem to decrease. Others, however, remain at a loss to cope with these anxieties.

Even women who thought they had released their fears simply by confessing them frequently continue to experience frightening nightmares. These expectant mothers apparently deny the existence of a reservoir of unexpressed emotions. In turn, constantly growing stress can cause high blood pressure, tension headaches, insomnia, or other stress symptoms. This type of denial and repression often evokes postpartum comments such as the ones below, collected by the San Francisco *Chronicle*'s roving reporter, the "Question Man":

A 40-year-old domestic engineer: The worst [part of the delivery] was the fear. They teach you how to breathe with the pain. That went out the window once the labor and the fear started.

A 36-year-old homemaker, mother of two: [The pregnancy] was always horrible. The best part was when it was over.

A 35-year-old research analyst: My least favorite thing was the last month. You're just so anxious to get it over with.

How much better to rid oneself of negativity and fear, so that after the baby's birth you can agree with these mothers, whose comments appeared in the same newspaper column:

A 32-year-old environmental scientist: I get a kick out of the movement of the baby. I just like the feeling of life inside.

A 30-year-old legal secretary: I loved the baby growing inside of me, first the butterflies and then when it really gets moving. You feel life being created and it gets your mind going.

These students, too, had resolved their fears:

Deborah, 33-year-old attorney: The labor was hard work but it was worth it. When my baby's head began to come out it was the most incredible feeling. The astronauts maybe felt a little that way when they first stepped onto the moon.

Lizette, 28-year-old sportswear buyer: I was prepared, but nobody can really tell you what it (labor) feels like. The power of the contractions surprised me. Also, it was definitely sexual, especially the relief when they let me bear down. Oh, there was some pain, yet it was not what I expected; more like the extreme effort that goes into an athletic event (running a marathon) than it was painful. For a few moments I felt a little panic and tensed up. Only then, for a short time, it really hurt, until my husband persuaded me to relax. All in all, we both agree it was the highest experience of our lives.

This last part of the book reinforces your ability to identify any repressed fears. Here, we review two methods. The first involves interpretation of the typical symbols, themes, patterns, and levels of dreams indicating fear. The second method depends on recognition of physical changes during painful, angry, or fearful experiences.

We also will reiterate and practice these techniques for coping with anxiety:

- Deep relaxation
- Incubating dreams and creating lucid dreams
- Reversing negative thoughts into positive ones
- Creating affirmations and positive daydreams

Additionally, the following chapters provide information and suggest resources for helping you to make safe, logical choices about the resolution of the problems or conflicts that cause anxiety. With this goal in mind, we will examine each major fear again and discuss the ways other pregnant women have dealt with them.

Anxiety-Provoking Myths

Modern technology has made obstetrics a safer and more exact science than ever before. Still, my research revealed a rising anxiety level among pregnant women, owing to misinformation about the risks of childbirth over age thirty; the dangers of prenatal tests; and the baby's need for a nonworking mother.

PREGNANCY AFTER THIRTY

The average childbearing age in America has changed in recent years, so that more women over thirty are now having babies than in previous generations. The following myths—all of them *false*—confront these mothers-to-be:

- Women over thirty nearly always have difficulty conceiving.
- Older women are more likely to have complicated deliveries and C-sections.

- Children of women over thirty are more likely to be malformed.
- Prenatal tests are very risky and often cause miscarriage.

Responding to the first issue, Lamaze authority Elizabeth Bing and psychologist Libby Colman, authors of *Having a Baby After 30,* say that while fertility does decline in both men and women with age, healthy couples over thirty can—and usually do—conceive without problems.

The follicles that eventually become eggs or ova are present in the female at birth. They mature during puberty, and continue to be released until menopause. Although fewer eggs are produced as age increases—so that some women in their thirties may not ovulate each month—most females have enough for conception until well into their forties.

Dr. Robert Nachtigall, gynecologist and fertility specialist at San Francisco's Children's Hospital, says that many cases of infertility result from anxiety. Many over-thirty couples feel pressured by time and fear that they're approaching unfertile years. When they stop using contraceptives but do not conceive immediately, they become needlessly anxious. This tension can interfere with women's ovulation and cause lower sperm counts in men.

Prolonged use of the pill or an intrauterine device (IUD) also may give rise to some conception problems. Many doctors advise discontinuing the pill for several months before trying to conceive. While the IUD has been suspected of causing fertility problems, statistics on the topic are unreliable.

Sometimes, advancing age also increases the likelihood that there may have been trauma or minor damage to your uterus, ovaries, or fallopian tubes. Simple tests usually can determine this, and the appropriate corrective measures can be done right in your physician's office with very little discomfort.

As to complicated pregnancies, I must reiterate the dangers of toxemia. Its symptoms include high blood pressure, swelling of the hands and feet due to water retention, weight gain after the twentieth week (again due to water retention), and too much protein in the urine. Your physician will routinely check for these symptoms. However, unless diabetic or carrying more than one fetus, you are less likely to experience toxemia symptoms than very young women under sixteen.

About twenty-five to thirty percent of all C-sections are among older women. Still, this statistic is misleading because it includes those whose previous pregnancies have left their abdominal muscles too stretched for successful labor or those who have developed other medical problems. If you remain in good health and follow a proper diet and exercise regimen, your chances of having a C-section should not be any higher than for women under thirty.

Recent studies reported in obstetrics periodicals such as *Birth* and the *ICEA Journal,* published by the International Childbirth Educators Association, nevertheless claim that some physicians tend to perform C-sections on healthy, first-time pregnant women over thirty. These practitioners tend to view their patients in the same light as older women who have had a number of children already.

If you are over thirty, ask your doctor and hospital personnel about their policy regarding C-sections. Especially pay attention to the rate of such operations performed in the past year. If you want a normal, vaginal delivery, make this quite clear to your physician.

A word of caution: some women, regardless of their age, have pelvic structures too small for the baby to emerge. In these cases, a C-section must be done. If your doctor says you may have such a condition, it's often advisable to experience some normal labor prior to the C-section, because the contractions massage the baby, possibly preventing respiratory problems after birth. Ask your physician about this procedure. Also remember to continue attending childbirth preparation classes with your husband; the course will provide information about measures enabling at least one of you to hold your baby upon delivery and helping you both recover rapidly from the operation.

Should you need a C-section, your childbirth instructor will tell you about the advantages this operation offers for the baby. These include less stress on the infant's heart and a smaller likelihood of certain birth defects occasionally resulting from an extremely prolonged labor.

Sometimes couples over forty have defective chromosomes in the ovum or the sperm. When these conditions are severe, the fetus usually will abort spontaneously. Milder defects often can be corrected either during your pregnancy or immediately after delivery. Couples with such problems also may have perfectly normal sperm and ova the next time they try to conceive. At present, the only way such defects can be diagnosed is after conception, although a genetics specialist is able to predict the likelihood of problems occurring in couples over forty. Generally, women from the ages of thirty to thirty-nine need not worry about abnormalities.

One of the most feared and perhaps overly publicized of fetal defects is Down's syndrome, commonly called mongolism. Although the chances of a baby's affliction increase with maternal age, what you read or hear is often misleading.

Bing and Colman state that the rate of Down's syndrome in women between thirty and thirty-four is only one in 750 births. The rate jumps sharply at age thirty-nine to one in 280 births and to one in 130 for mothers between forty and forty-four. One in 65 babies born to women over forty-five will have Down's syndrome. In other words, if you are under 35, the chances of your baby being affected are quite small.

Women in their forties should consult a genetics specialist before conceiving to get a prediction of the possible outcome for self and partner as individuals. The practitioner takes into account your specific medical history; therefore, you won't be forced to rely on general statements by the press. If already pregnant at this age, you should take tests to determine the health of your baby. Some abnormalities can be corrected before the infant is born. In other instances, tests prepare physicians so that the baby can be treated immediately after delivery.

Physicians may recommend amniocentesis for women between thirty-five and forty to determine if the fetus is likely to have Down's syndrome. This test also reveals other possible abnormalities.

PRENATAL TESTS

In addition, a number of prenatal tests can tell you how your pregnancy is progressing and can determine certain physiological aspects of your unborn child. Some of these tests are so new, however, that all possible side effects have not been evaluated. With the exception of the AFP (a safe, simple blood test), no test should be taken just out of curiosity. Furthermore, certain ones are slightly risky. These should be done only if other, safer tests indicate the need. The following is a list of the most commonly used prenatal tests:

First- and second-trimester tests
Ultrasound (Sonogram)
Alpha Fetaprotein Screening (AFP)
Chorionic Villi Sampling (CVS)
Amniocentesis

Third-trimester tests
Fetal Movement Monitoring
Fetal Biophysical Profile
Non-Stress Test
Contraction Stress Test

Ultrasound (Sonogram). A machine something like your dentist's x-ray equipment bounces high-frequency sound waves off the fetus. These change according to the density of the objects through which they pass.

This test can tell you how far along in your pregnancy you are; the possible causes of any vaginal bleeding; whether you are carrying more than one fetus; whether the sac contains the right amount of amniotic fluid; the condition of the placenta; how the baby is growing; and whether any major fetal defects exist. If the display screen happens to show your fetus in profile, you may be able to tell its sex. Again, curiosity does not provide sufficient reason for you to undergo ultrasound testing. Although it has been in use for twenty-five years without showing convincing evidence of dangerous side effects, we remain uncertain as to whether ultrasound may cause long-term harm to the fetus.

Alpha fetaprotein screening (AFP). This simple procedure, safe as any other blood test, shows abnormalities of the fetal spinal cord and abdominal wall. Usually, these defects can be corrected by simple surgery on the baby immediately after birth. The only disadvantage of the AFP test is that the findings of abnormality may not be accurate. Therefore, other examinations probably will have to be done to confirm its results.

Chorionic villi sampling (CVS). Similar to amniocentesis, this test is done at an earlier stage of pregnancy, between the eighth and twelfth week. It screens women over thirty-five and others who have special medical problems such as diabetes. Using a syringe or hollow tube, the physician removes some of the tissue surrounding the fetus.

CVS reveals fetal abnormalities sooner than amniocentesis, allowing couples to make the decision to abort at an earlier and safer date. On the other hand, the test has definitely been shown to cause miscarriage in one out of 200 women, and recent studies indicate a potentially higher rate. Couples who have a history of miscarriages or who had difficulty conceiving may not want to risk CVS. Also, because its results are not conclusive, women who take the test may still have to undergo amniocentesis.

Amniocentesis. This test involves inserting a needle in the abdomen to remove about three tablespoons of the amniotic fluid surrounding the fetus. This liquid contains cells shed by the developing child, so that laboratory technicians can determine if your baby has Down's syndrome or other hereditary disorders. Amniocentesis also may show the infant's sex, although in some cases the gender information is not accurate. The test is not performed until the fifteenth to seventeenth week of pregnancy.

Amniocentesis results take several weeks to process; thus, if you decide to abort, the risks are greater than they would have been with the CVS test. Additionally, miscarriages do occur because of amniocentesis, although the rate remains lower than one in 200.

The last four tests on my list are not usually done unless complications develop during the last trimester. These procedures then help physicians to decide whether the mother should deliver prematurely or let the fetus remain in her uterus full-term. While other tests sometimes become necessary if complications arise, the following third-trimester tests are the most common:

Fetal movement monitoring. You perform this test yourself by counting the number of times the fetus moves in a thirty- or sixty-minute period. If it does not move more than ten times an hour, or not at all for twelve hours, you should take further tests to determine the baby's condition.

Fetal biophysical profile. The doctor performs this test with a very advanced type of ultrasound scanner, giving the baby what amounts to a complete physical exam. Breathing, muscle tone, movement, and amniotic fluid are all examined. If the test indicates low oxygen supply, the fetus could be in distress and your doctor may advise premature delivery.

Non-Stress test. In some hospitals this test is used routinely, so if it is done while you're in labor there's no need for alarm. A nonbinding strap is put around your belly to hold an external fetal monitor. This measures the fetal heart rate, which normally speeds up when the fetus moves. Two such increases in heart rate every twenty minutes mean that your baby is healthy.

Contraction stress test. To determine how well the fetus will be able to endure the stress of contractions, labor is induced by stimulating the mother's nipples or by intravenously injecting oxytocin, a contraction-inducing hormone. The fetal heart rate is then measured to determine if any problems may develop during delivery.

Controversy surrounds this test—and administration of oxytocin—because the painful contractions that result require sedation of the mother, in turn presenting risks to the fetus. This test probably should not be done unless life-threatening complications exist.

Some physicians also administer oxytocin to induce labor when the pregnancy is well past the due date. Again, we advise against this procedure unless other complications present themselves. According to childbirth educator Carl Jones, it's usually far better to trigger labor by biking or jogging, eating spicy foods, or drinking carbonated beverages. Jones says that overly active intestines often bring on a very late labor. However, be sure to check with your doctor or midwife before trying any of these suggestions.

EFFECTS ON YOUR BABY WHEN YOU WORK

Nowadays we hear a great deal about the psychological importance of close, constant contact (bonding) between the parents and the newborn as soon after birth as possible, in addition to the beneficial physical effects of breast milk. These issues came to the fore in 1977, when the American Medical Association issued a bulletin to all obstetrical personnel stating the necessity for both baby and parents to have this skin-to-skin and eye-to-eye contact. Physicians and hospitals subsequently have made bonding more practical and convenient by including expectant fathers in delivery rooms and installing alternative birthing centers and "lying-in" arrangements so that babies need not be taken to nurseries while their mothers recover.

Some parents translate bonding into a belief that the babies of working mothers will not develop normally; this may give rise to agonizing conflicts during pregnancy. However, careful planning can insure your baby's emotional and physical well-being and normal growth, whether you stay at home or return to work.

If you and/or the baby's father bond with your infant as soon after birth as possible, and if the main caregiver holds your newborn frequently and provides plenty of cuddling and rocking, the child need not suffer if you return to work. If you're convinced that you should nurse your baby, you can get off to a good start while you're on maternity leave. Upon returning to work, you can express your milk every evening or morning, freeze it, and it can be fed by bottle to your baby in your absence. Today, thousands of American mothers work and raise happy, well-adjusted, and healthy children.

Now that we've examined the myths that frequently give rise to needless anxiety, let's see how they form the basis for the six major fears experienced during pregnancy; how these anxieties are reflected in your dreams; and how you can cope with them.

CHAPTER 9

❖

Dreams that Your Baby Will Be Deformed or Die

The fear that there may be something wrong with the unborn child probably haunts every expectant parent. While mothers-to-be may have struggled with this fear for centuries, it appears to be more widespread now because many contemporary pregnant women are older. For example, in her fourth month, 32-year-old Frances reported:

> I dreamed I was in the hospital having my baby. I was in an operating room. The doctor told me to push and a nurse told me to bear down. I did and then the doctor held up a tiny wet baby kitten. He said, "It's a boy—and here comes another one!" I grunted and looked down. Another tiny kitten popped out of me. Then another and one more. There were four or five. I lost count. They started crawling all over my stomach and my breasts and sucking at my nipples. I wasn't upset at all. I was happy, and thought they were really cute and I was petting them. (Then I woke up and felt scared, thinking this might mean there's something wrong with my baby.)

Dreams of Animals

When Frances discovered that hundreds of pregnant women share this type of dream and that the kittens probably represented the fetus and happy feelings about her unborn child, she was quite relieved. Such dreams may seem amusing or bizarre to the nonpregnant, but they are not funny at all to the mother-to-be, already so fearful of the myths and misconceptions mentioned earlier. Then, when they have dreams of giving birth to small animals, their worries may increase.

Lilah, a 31-year-old secretary, had this dream in her fifth month:

> I am in the maternity ward, and already had my baby. A nurse brings it to me all wrapped in receiving blankets. When I open up the blankets, there's a puppy inside. I yell for the nurse who returns. "This is not my baby!" I tell her. She says, "Oh, yes it is. See the ID bracelet on him? It's yours, all right." And she leaves. Then I notice all the other women in the ward have little puppies in their arms. (I woke up feeling guilty and worried that something's wrong with my baby.)

Lilah's dream was unusual in that it occurred so late in her pregnancy; dreams of small animals more typically crop up during the first and second trimesters. Also, unlike Lilah, most mothers appear happy in these dreams of giving birth to adorable little animals, usually experiencing fear only after they awaken.

When we discussed her feelings, Lilah told us this was an unplanned pregnancy. "In the first two months," she said, "I even tried to make myself miscarry by doing strenuous exercise, drinking a bit more than usual, taking laxatives. Then Ben [her husband] and I talked it over because he wanted me to have it. We even went to a marriage counselor. Finally, I agreed to have the baby. Guess I'm still not completely glad about it. Also," she continued, "I do feel guilty, afraid something I might have done early on may have hurt the fetus."

Although she appeared to be more accepting of her pregnancy after participating in my relaxation classes, Lilah continued to have nightmarish dreams right up until her delivery. She returned to our reunion class with her healthy baby girl, and told us, "I can't believe I was so negative about having her! I love her so much, and as soon as the doctor says it's okay, I want to have another!"

Once they understand that dreams of small animals are typical of early pregnancy, most women begin to enjoy them. However, mothers-to-be sometimes cannot comprehend how large or threatening animals could possibly symbolize the unborn child. The following are some excerpts from this type of dream:

> *Bertie, 25-year-old nurse in her sixth month:* Leaving the hospital at 2 A.M., I was startled by a huge black bear which came lumbering out of the bushes behind the parking lot. . . . I jumped in my car and it followed, roaring at me.

> *Eve, 28-year-old supermarket checker, in her seventh month:* We were vacationing at a camp in the woods . . . there were some hideous devil dogs outside. . . . Very scary.

> *Marcia, 32-year-old homemaker in her second pregnancy:* This big, wild dog jumped up from the back seat . . . more like a wolf . . . fangs dripped blood . . . about to attack my son.

These dreams of overwhelming or threatening animals generally occur during the last trimester. As the expectant mother's abdomen becomes larger and she feels clumsy, awkward, and occasionally at the mercy of her condition, it's quite natural for her to resent being pregnant or to be impatient for the end. As a result, these feelings sometimes reveal themselves in dreams portraying menacing fetal or pregnancy symbols.

Bertie was becoming overly fatigued by continuing to work on a night shift until her scheduled maternity leave.

She thought the huge black bear symbolized both her feelings about the fetus and about her job, which she feared threatened her health. "I didn't admit it until I had this dream," she said. "Then I told my supervisor I either had to take early leave or go onto a day shift, part-time."

Eve was worried that something might be wrong with her baby because she thought the "devil dogs" represented the fetus. Out of context, this might seem to be true; however, the remainder of Eve's nightmare described her husband's leaving the safety of the lodge to hunt down the menacing dogs and reports from other dream characters that he had been killed. The monsters thus seemed to reflect her fear of losing her mate more than they did her fear of carrying an unhealthy baby. This raises a good point: always examine your own associations to any dream symbol rather than unquestioningly accepting any standard meaning.

Marcia's nightmare of the attacking "wolf dog" is more typical than the other dream animals, because Marcia was unconsciously worried about the relationship between the new baby and her son. Women who have other children more frequently envision large, threatening creatures than do first-time moms.

Different dreams about the well-being of the unborn child often seem more disturbing than those featuring animals. Usually nightmarish in quality, they appear to reflect the dreamer's fear that the baby will be born deformed, diseased, or even dead.

Dreams of Harm to the Fetus

Anxiety about an infant's health often yields the most frightening dreams. For instance, Portia, a 35-year-old homemaker, had the following nightmare in her second trimester:

> Dreamed I was at the meat counter in the supermarket. A
> clerk, who looked exactly like my obstetrician, invited me

to come around behind the counter to pick out what I wanted. We went into this refrigerated room where all kinds of carcasses were hanging. I felt horrified at this bloody sight. On one side was a string of small ones. I asked what they were and he grinned and said, "Those are human babies that were defective or dead. They're delicious but we usually don't tell customers what they are. Want to try one?" I felt scared and sick (and woke up really terrified).

Portia had undergone amniocentesis a few days before this dream and her doctor assured her of a normal fetus. Nevertheless, she continued to worry, both that her baby might have some defects and that the test might cause her to miscarry.

Both these fears surfaced in her dream, with the clerk so obviously resembling her physician, and his telling her that the smaller carcasses were babies. To help Portia confront her irrational fears, I taught her to create the sort of positive daydreams and affirmations that could be integrated into her deeper consciousness each night when she relaxed.

As it turned out, Portia had to have a C-section: after eighteen hours of labor, the fetal monitors showed her baby in distress, with an abnormal heart beat. The seven-pound, four-ounce boy proved to be healthy, however, and Portia brought the baby to our class reunion. She told us, "My labor may have been so long because I had trouble relaxing. The truth is, I just did not practice doing the relaxation exercises or the daydreams, especially in my last trimester. Next time, I'll know better. Anyhow, my baby's fine and I've recovered, so it all had a happy ending."

Rosemary's Baby Dreams

Dream researcher Dr. Robert Van de Castle speculates that "Rosemary's Baby" dreams reflect the pregnant woman's feeling that her body has been invaded by something ugly or dangerous.

Even well-informed women who planned their pregnancies occasionally admit these feelings. "I had no idea I'd feel so repulsed about my body," confessed Brenda, a 33-year-old pediatric nurse in her first pregnancy. "Even though my head tells me what's going on inside my belly, sometimes I feel as if I'm carrying something alien or gross, like a tumor or cancer."

In her second trimester, Brenda dreamed that her baby was born with an adult appearance:

> I was in labor and my husband went out to go to the restroom. I had begged him to wait but he went anyway. I knew that the baby was coming fast and I was scared to deliver alone. But I looked down and there, sitting between my legs, was this naked little boy about the size of a three- or four-year-old. He looked like a little cherub with blond curls. Then as I looked more closely I saw his face was like an old man's and there were fangs coming out of his lips. I said, "We're supposed to bond, so come up here and give me a hug." But he stood up and started jumping up and down on my stomach. . . . He jumped hard on my stomach and it hurt. I started to scream and he just gave me this evil look and kept on, like he was on a trampoline. (I woke up shaking and crying and my husband said I'd been groaning in my sleep.)

Brenda's worry that the baby might be defective is symbolized by its evil, devilish appearance. Her other fears—her husband's lack of support during labor, and her own inability to care for a newborn—also are depicted in this dream.

"Everybody assumes that, because I'm a nurse and specialize in child care, I'll just sail through labor and mothering a newborn with no problems," Brenda explained. "But actually, I'm just as scared as any other new mother and I want my husband to be there. Also, I know the basics, of course, about caring for the newborn. But in my work I deal with older children mostly, so I do get a little worried about taking care of a tiny infant, too. That's probably why I dreamed about a toddler instead of a small baby."

Usually, ambivalent feelings about your pregnancy or your baby simply mean that you have not yet reached the emotional stage of what Dr. Helene Deutsch in *The Psychology of Women* describes as "incorporation of the fetus." At that time, the mother-to-be no longer views pregnancy as an invasion; the baby now is a part of her. Expectant women generally "incorporate the baby" by the third trimester.

More important, however, you must avoid anxiety and be as relaxed as possible throughout your pregnancy. If your dreams are nightmarish, the underlying fears should be dispelled. Also, feelings of body invasion persisting into the third trimester ought to be confronted at a deeper level of consciousness. In addition to making you feel more comfortable for the rest of your pregnancy, this acceptance may also be important to your baby's emotional development. There is increasing support for the theory that the unborn child may be aware of its mother's feelings. Much talk nowadays focuses on "intrauterine bonding," the communication of loving thoughts and feelings to the unborn.

Although strict scientific evidence does not support this New Age idea, it has been established that well-adjusted pregnant women give birth to happy, contented babies. For these reasons, negative thoughts about your baby's health and your acceptance of your pregnancy should be replaced by positive and nourishing attitudes.

Coping with Negativity About Your Pregnancy and Your Baby

There are several ways you can cope with needless fear so that you can relax as you should while awaiting your delivery. These include

- Understanding the source of your fears
- Informing yourself about actual risks
- Practicing deep relaxation regularly
- Creating positive affirmations and daydreams
- Incubating dreams and dreaming lucidly

WHY ARE YOU TENSE OR ANXIOUS?

Now is the time to check your body for physical signs of anxiety or tension. You may wish to review Chapter 5 on understanding your emotions to refresh your memory about the symptoms of unexpressed fear.

If you are experiencing a more rapid heartbeat than usual, rapid or shallow breathing, cool or cold perspiration, then anxiety has surfaced. Tight muscles, especially in your throat or chest, also usually indicate repressed worries. Other signs of tension caused by unexpressed anxiety may include headaches, nausea, dizziness, trembling, or merely an overall feeling of dread.

As with all the other major pregnancy anxieties, the first step in coping with concerns about your baby's health is to identify their source. If your dreams reflect concern about your unborn child's well-being, similar to Lilah's dream of giving birth to a puppy, then it's highly likely that you do have this unexpressed anxiety about your baby or your pregnancy. It's natural and normal to have at least some fleeting thoughts about complicated labor or other unknown factors that may affect the baby's health. In fact, if you and your partner exhibit no worries, you are rare indeed!

INFORMING YOURSELF

Once you have identified the cause of your concern, the next step is to inform yourself about the likelihood of any risks to your baby. As the beginning of Chapter 8 emphasizes, even if you're over thirty, the medical hazards are considerably less than they were a generation ago. Stillbirths or deformed babies are actually quite uncommon.

When it's right to worry. Although most fears regarding the baby's health are needless, valid reasons for concern do exist. If you drink alcohol, smoke, or use recreational drugs, you should be very worried about your infant's health. Stop right now! If you find yourself unable to quit, please don't blame yourself or feel overly guilty. Instead, consult the yellow pages for self-help groups or private counseling, and get busy making yourself as healthy as possible for your own and your baby's sake. If you used these substances in the past, be sure to inform your doctor so that she or he can be on the alert for symptoms.

Utilizing resources. In addition to reading this book, you can investigate other sources of information. Check the yellow pages, hospitals, or your local chapter of the International Childbirth Educators Association (ICEA) for early pregnancy courses. If some specific item about your own or your baby's health worries you and you are not enrolled in such a class, your doctor and/or midwife will probably be happy to answer your questions.

Furthermore, unless you're a substance abuser or over thirty-five, there's usually little cause for concern if your medical check-ups show no complications. With all these reassurances, it's time to let go of such fears. Then, you may be pleasantly surprised to find that your dreams appear to be helping rather than frightening you.

Jennifer was a generally well-adjusted, self-confident young woman expecting her first child. Like many of the volunteers for my doctoral research, she claimed to have no worries and to be looking forward to childbirth with pleasure. However, she would always add, "Of course I do wonder if the baby's okay. You know, if it has all its fingers and toes, that sort of thing."

At my suggestion, Jennifer thoroughly informed herself about the possible risks of such deformities. Then in her sixth month, she dreamed:

> I could distinctly feel the shape, size, and number of toes of our baby's foot. I remember dreaming that I said to my husband and Mom to feel the foot. It was such a neat feeling it is hard to describe.

Another dream followed that same night:

> My whole stomach was transparent and I could see and
> feel the whole baby's body, except to tell if it was a boy
> or girl. It was really something!

Obviously, Jennifer's dreaming self took very seriously—
and literally—her expressed concern about whether the
baby would have all its fingers and toes. Then, perhaps to
totally convince herself, she dreamed of actually viewing her
unborn child in the womb.

Jennifer's experience was not very typical, however. Even
when reason dictates no need for worry, many expectant
parents nevertheless find themselves plagued with negative
thoughts and nightmares about the possibility of infant disease, deformity, or stillbirth. If you're one of these, now is
the time to make use of your new knowledge of the powers
of your mind to dispel your fears.

USING YOUR MIND'S POWERS TO CONQUER FEAR

If you have practiced the steps outlined in the second part
of this book, you already may know how amazingly powerful your dreams and your right-brain abilities can be.
Dreams often help you identify unexpressed fears and other
emotions as well as provide solutions to the conflicts and
problems of your waking life.

By getting in touch with your right-brain abilities, you
can envision situations and attitudes which will, in fact,
become realities once integrated into your deeper consciousness. However, none of these powers is readily available
unless you have learned sound relaxation practices.

You now may wish to review Chapter 3 and its directions
for deep relaxation. Then, find a quiet, private place and a
time when you won't be distracted, breathe deeply, and
listen to your relaxation tape (or your partner) for instructions. Once in that wonderfully restful state, "limp as a

dishrag," focus on your creative daydream, either by reviewing your tape or your dream diary entry.

Lilah created the following after having dreamed of giving birth to a puppy:

> I am in the maternity ward and the nurse brings my baby, wrapped in receiving blankets. I open them and there is my beautiful, tiny new little girl. The nurse helps me diaper her and change her little shirt. Then I'm able to see that every part of her is perfect. I put her to my breast and she sucks greedily. Even though I don't have any milk yet, the nurse explains that the cholostrum which is coming out is important to help my daughter develop immunities. I love her so much. My husband comes in and sits beside us. He whispers, "The other babies in this ward are cute—but I think ours is the prettiest of all!"

After she relaxed and integrated this daydream one quiet afternoon, a remarkable thing happened to Lilah. That night, she had an almost identical dream. It was as if she were telling herself that she had, indeed, let go of her fear that something might be wrong with her unborn child.

If you keep informed about the minimal risks of childbirth, practice deep relaxation and creative daydreaming, and still experience nightmares about your baby's well-being, check your own health habits. Take every possible precaution—including proper nutrition, exercise, and regular examinations with your midwife or physician.

Suppose your inner self still fails to yield positive dreams of your unborn? Review Chapter 7 and incubate a dream that will show you your baby. If your baby previously was depicted as defective in some manner, it becomes even more important to follow this technique and get a true picture of the fetus.

After her nightmare about the threatening black bear, the nurse Bertie incubated a dream by relaxing deeply and then repeating to herself over and over until she fell asleep, "I will dream about my baby tonight." A few hours later, the following dream resulted:

> The same big black bear came out of the bushes. This time, it picked me up and carried me to a kind of shack the hospital gardeners use. I felt very frightened. (I woke up and stayed there very still with my eyes closed, thinking this was not the kind of dream I had hoped to have. Then I thought I'd just try to go back into it and see what would happen, so I went back to sleep.) Now it was like a rerun of an old movie! The bear came out of the bushes again, grabbed me, and took me to that same old shack. (I don't know if this was what you call a lucid type of dream, since I don't remember knowing I was dreaming at the time. Yet it might have been, since I sort of directed things after that.) Then I tried to be calm and I told the bear very firmly to put me down. He did, onto a chair in the shack. He was huge and dark brown, almost black. I looked up and said, "Now just what do you want with me?" And he kind of kneeled down and put that big shaggy head in my lap. I said, "I don't mean to hurt your feelings, but I wanted to see my baby, not you." Then he lifted his shaggy face off like a mask with one big paw and underneath was a real, live baby! I just stared and stared at it and it smiled and made baby gurgling sounds at me. (Then I woke up feeling so happy I was almost laughing out loud!)

Bertie is similar to her professional peers. One might think medical personnel would be less fearful because of their education, yet they are often even more anxious about their own pregnancies than less experienced women. This possibly happens because professionals see rare cases and serious complications.

Many women who already have had children frequently share similar anxieties, usually because their previous pregnancies and deliveries were difficult. Therefore, I urge you to attend childbirth preparation classes, even if you believe you're well informed. In these classes you can share your worries with others like yourself, question your fears, and find out the most recent advances in obstetrical technology.

If either your spontaneous or incubated dreams continue to depict an unhealthy baby after taking all these precautions, you still cannot rule out the possibility of negative attitudes. This is the ideal time to practice more deep relaxation, followed by the integration of affirmations (see the Appendix).

Finally, tell yourself on a daily basis that 98 out of 100 babies born in the United States are normal. The statistical probability remains highly skewed toward your side. If you are healthy and reasonably conscientious, you will take pleasure in bringing to life the perfect child you anticipate.

Don't be afraid to unmask your fears. Keep in mind the subtle yet dangerous effects of unexpressed anxiety, and resolve to face this particular concern, here and now. Search your mind and dreams for any lingering negativity that may keep you from relaxing. Trust your body and the creative energy within to nurture your baby as it grows, developing normally day-by-day.

CHAPTER 10

❖

Dreams of Being an Inadequate Parent

If you plan to work after the baby comes, you may be worried about how your absence will affect the baby, finding good day care, and what measures you'll be able to take should you have to miss work to care for the baby. If you have other children, you'll probably have some anxiety about being able to care for a larger family, as well as about the possibility of sibling rivalry. If this is your first pregnancy, you may feel unsure about your ability to give your baby the proper care.

All these worries are normal, evidence that you love both your unborn child and your family. What's important is to learn to identify these concerns so that you can take steps to dispel them. Your dreams should be the first discovery point.

Have you dreamed of being unable to protect or care for plants or small animals, likely fetal symbols? In the fourth month of her first pregnancy, 24-year-old Amelia, a part-time secretary, reported this episode:

I dreamed I was watering and weeding our vegetable garden. For some reason, I couldn't seem to get hold of anything. I kept dropping the hose. One vine had a big squash on it that was growing bigger right there as I watched! The squash was covered with bugs and I couldn't get them off. I took off my garden gloves and saw that each hand had five thumbs and no fingers. I just squatted there and cried and cried—more about the squash than about my hands. Feeling real grief because I couldn't take care of it and the bugs were ruining it. (When I woke up I was actually shaking with fear and sadness, too.)

Dreams of Botanical Images

Botanical images such as plants, flowers, fruits, and vegetables are frequent fetal symbols in first trimester dreams. These representations of the growing life within often change to larger plants, trees, and even vast, overgrown jungles as the pregnancy progresses.

Amelia saw that her dream quite literally indicated fears of being "all thumbs" in caring for a newborn. The squash, she agreed, symbolized her pregnancy and the fetus. Just as she appeared unable to keep the bugs from ruining her dream plants, Amelia feared her inexperience would endanger her baby's health after it was born.

Many contemporary pregnant women share Amelia's self-image: being inadequate, clumsy, and incapable of caring for a tiny infant. Usually this anxiety arises because today's mothers-to-be have not grown up in large families or in a time when teenagers watched over the infants who are now in day care facilities.

Further, more expectant women are older and working today than ever before, a circumstance often preventing them from being in contact with neighborhood parents and children as might have been the case generations ago.

Contemporary pregnant women's dreams often reflect

this anxiety. The following provide good—and typical— examples:

> *Betty Anne, 22-year-old graduate student in her third month:* Overwatered all Mom's house plants . . . she came home and was furious . . . "If you didn't know how, you should've found out!" she scolded.

> *Stefanie, 30-year-old bakery chef in her fourth month:* Got to work after lunch to find the hanging plants in the salesroom had dripped all over the bread and the little gingerbread boy cookies . . . had to bake them all over again. . . . Then couldn't remove the plant . . . it had grown to double its size.

> *Serena, 34-year-old attorney in her seventh month:* A long dream . . . began in a choppy river in a jungle . . . after we capsized I had to walk barefoot on a muddy path, very dangerous. . . . Our guide gave me a machete, but I couldn't keep the heavy vines away. They seemed like live animals, grasping at me. . . . (Woke up screaming and my husband was disturbed and upset with all my racket.)

These excerpts, filled with common botanical images, emphasize women's fears of being unable to care for the baby to come. This worry is frequently compounded by doubts about competently juggling career and parental duties.

Betty Anne's dreams of not being able to care for her mother's plants was similar to Amelia's dreams of clumsiness: both women saw the greenery as fetal symbols they were unable to nurture.

Envisioning dripping plants ruining her baked goods (specifically, gingerbread boys), Stephanie also worried that she could not care for her baby. Her dream also depicts the career-versus-motherhood conflict.

Serena's dream also richly symbolized her stage of pregnancy and anxiety about being an adequate mother. The choppy river waters represent approaching labor and the capsized boat, a difficult delivery. Instead of house plants, this third trimester dream is replete with lush jungle growth and animated vines—fetal symbols evading Serena's powers of control. This anxiety about being a competent parent occurs in many women's dreams throughout pregnancy and usually takes the form of a fetal symbol being harmed, threatened, or inadequately cared for by the dreamer or a mother figure.

Dreams of Small Children

Some psychologists, including Van de Castle and Deutsch, say that when pregnant women dream of toddlers or small children—and especially of giving birth to them—this probably indicates the expectant mother's wish to avoid the difficulties of tending to a tiny infant. In other words, these experts again believe such dreams portray fears of being an inadequate parent.

However, Dr. Cecilia Jones, who studied thirteen subjects during their first pregnancies, theorized that older babies might represent the women when they were children, rather than the fetus. My own research attempted to find out what the dreamers thought these child characters symbolized. Here are some excerpts:

> *Chelsea, 27-year-old waitress in her fifth month:* I saw a little girl about two or three on a seesaw with her father weighing down one end . . . he bumped her off . . . her mother wasn't even watching.

> *Lira, 33-year-old lab technician in her eighth month:* My baby just slipped out of me onto my bed . . . so easy. . . . He was sitting up, already diapered, so cute!

> *Bobbie, 22-year-old bookkeeper in her fifth month:* My Lamaze teacher was pushing a stroller with a little baby girl in it . . . looked like me . . . she slapped the child.

Chelsea thought her dream of the child on a seesaw did not represent her baby at all, but herself. As our discussion progressed, it developed that Chelsea's father had abused both her and her mother when she was a child, and she thought the dream recalled her feelings of those years before her mother finally divorced her father.

"It just makes me sick with rage and pain when I even hear about child abuse," she confided. "I've had a lot of therapy to help me. But I know I'll never, ever even spank my own children. I'll probably have trouble disciplining them at all, rather than the other way around." Chelsea also admitted to anxiety about "not being a good mother," because she had heard that adults who were abused as children tend to repeat their parents' behavior.

Lira, on the other hand, saw that her dream of delivering an older infant with such ease probably represented a wish to "just bypass both labor and taking care of a brand new baby."

In our study group, Bobbie decided the Lamaze instructor in her dream portrayed her own mother's parenting style. "She wasn't really abusive," Bobbie explained. "It was more that she was overworked, and when she got tired she'd lose her temper. But she'd always tell us kids how sorry she was, and we knew how much she loved us." Nevertheless, Bobbie vowed she would quit work after her baby came, rather than allow herself to become overly fatigued and cross with her own children.

By disguising the parent figure in the dream and presenting her as a likable person (the Lamaze teacher), Bobbie's dreaming self might have been trying to reveal her tendency to defend her mother, denying that she had not been a loving parent.

Dreams of Animals

We've already discussed many early pregnancy dreams depicting small animals as fetal symbols. Any harm done to these little creatures often indicates an anxiety about being an adequate parent.

Later pregnancy dreams also show this same fear, although the fetal symbols may be different. During the last trimester, women will sometimes see larger animals, rather than the small furry kittens, bunnies, or mice of the early months. For example, Holly, a 35-year-old expectant mother who raised poultry with her husband Walter, appeared troubled by a number of issues when she came to me for counseling. Her doctor had told her that her pelvis was too small, making her a likely candidate for a C-section. Although sonograms revealed no abnormalities, Holly worried about her baby's health as well. She reported this unusual dream in her third trimester:

> Walter and I were raising giant, six-foot-tall turkeys. One of their peculiar characteristics was that they liked to be near people, but only if the person approached them backwards. The turkeys would flap away in fright if anyone approached them head-on. Walter and I were experimenting with this by slowly walking toward a group of them and just averting our faces. But one hen turkey, the largest of all, ran away. It left a huge egg which was in the midst of hatching. The baby turkey's head came out and then the egg started to roll, in the direction of another giant male turkey. I was very upset, thinking the male would eat the baby because it was pecking at it. But the egg kept rolling. But it was too late, the baby had been damaged. It hatched but began to die. We stood there horrified, not knowing what to do. (I began to cry and woke up.)

Holly and I spent almost an hour interpreting this bizarre nightmare. It's obvious that the dream reflects many concerns, such as Holly's fear of the fetus being too large for her small pelvis. Additionally, the large turkeys that needed to be approached backwards may have indicated to her that the baby was in a breech position. This, in fact, proved to be the case when Holly's labor began.

As we discussed this dream, Holly admitted to concern

over her child suffering damage at birth, as well as her own inability to care for the infant—just as she found herself helpless with the baby turkey in her dream. "I didn't even know I was worried about that too, until now," she told me. "No wonder I've been so tense lately." At my suggestion, Holly and Walter began attending Bradley childbirth preparation classes, where the male instructor was able to help diminish most of their fears and give them hands-on practice caring for his own small baby.

Dreams of Harm to Siblings

If you already have a child or children, do fetal symbols such as small or large animals attack them? Marcia, a 32-year-old homemaker with an 8-year-old son, appeared especially troubled by this sort of nightmare. In her third trimester, she reported the following:

> I was in a parking lot with Johnny, my son, after a shopping trip for layette things. Johnny was very tired and cross and wanted me to carry him but I couldn't, being too pregnant and tired myself. When we got to our car, it had been broken into. A lot of packages I'd left in the back seat, new baby things, were gone. The seat was all ripped up like it had been clawed. We got in and as we started out of the lot this big, wild dog jumped up from the back seat, growling and snarling. He looked like he was about to attack Johnny. This dog was really scary, looked more like a wolf than a dog, with long fangs that dripped blood. I remember it had awful looking sores all over its head and neck. Johnny started screaming, terrified. I yelled at him to jump out of the car but he couldn't get the door open. I slammed on the brakes and that threw the animal off balance. Then I grabbed an umbrella off the floor and started beating him down. I punched him in the stomach. It suddenly erupted and all this vile yellowish stuff came out. Then some worms started crawling out of the yellow mess. I woke up. (This terrible dream was so realistic I woke up feeling sick and had to go throw up. It's the first

time I've been sick since I got pregnant, but it felt just like the morning sickness when I had my first. Only I'm in my eighth month, so it couldn't be that. It was evidently the dream, which seemed so real.)

You may recall the excerpt from this nightmare quoted earlier, pointing out Marcia's worries about the health of her unborn child. Seeing the entire dream, you now can try your skills at interpreting its many fetal and pregnancy symbols. For instance, the car (Marcia's body) appears laden with baby things (the fetus). This vehicle also has been invaded by the wolf dog (fetal symbol), now attacking Johnny. Marcia's fight with the animal may represent her perception of the upcoming delivery, since she recalled a difficult time when her son was born. However, the main theme of this nightmare is a fear that the new baby would make Johnny feel jealous and pushed aside.

Two other expectant mothers' dreams mirror similar fears:

Coco, 31-year-old homemaker, mother of two: The marigold seeds had grown overnight into a jungle . . . my two kids were in there crying. . . . I tried to cut back the growth but I couldn't.

Yvette, 35-year-old nursery school teacher, mother of an 18-month-old: At school, pumpkins we got to make jack-o-lanterns began to grow! The children were so excited. . . . I got into a panic when the kids wouldn't obey me and leave the room . . . the pumpkins became dangerous monsters.

Coco's dream of the marigolds becoming a jungle is a marvelous representation of the way small plants and fetal symbols grow larger as the pregnancy progresses. When she had this dream, Coco was nearing the end of her second trimester, the time when these symbols sometimes begin to expand with the enlarging abdomen. The dream is also typical of women who have other children; here, Coco fears that she won't be an adequate parent for three youngsters.

Yvette's dream reflects similar anxieties but differs in that the small children in her nursery school class represented both the unborn infant and her 18-month-old toddler. According to Yvette, the rapidly growing pumpkins symbolized her pregnancy and the fetus: she was only in her fourth month and already quite large. A later sonogram showed that she was carrying twins, who were born normally after a comparatively brief ten-hour labor.

MANAGING AN ADDITIONAL CHILD

As it turned out, Yvette told us she was finding it much less difficult to manage than she'd imagined. "After I joined a support group for mothers of twins," she explained, "I learned all kinds of helpful tricks. It's almost as if I had to take care of triplets for awhile, instead of twins, since my first was still in diapers when the twins were born. But it's okay, although I couldn't have done it without the group and my husband's support."

When Marcia, who dreamed of the wolf dog attacking her 8-year-old son, recognized her overly anxious state, she read everything she could find about sibling rivalry. She also gave Johnny some appealing children's books to help prepare him for the new baby.

Childbirth educators Sandra Van Dam Anderson and Penny Simkin, authors of *Birth—Through Children's Eyes,* suggest that older siblings should be allowed to be present or nearby during the delivery. When they understood how this might help their son, Marcia and her husband decided to look for an institution that permitted this. They found such a birthing center, Johnny was present, and Marcia reports that he seems to be adjusting quite well to his new baby sister—who is healthy after a normal, uncomplicated delivery.

Blanche, a 28-year-old beautician, also showed concern about sibling rivalry. She reported this dream about two weeks before her baby boy was born:

I dreamt it was my 2-year-old daughter Katy's birthday party. I had already had the baby and he was fussing all during the party. All these other 2- and 3-year-olds were there and going wild, throwing cake and ice cream all over the living room. One of the littlest ones threw a block and hit Katy in the face, making her nose bleed. I felt relieved when some of the mothers came to pick them up. One was my next-door neighbor, who is also pregnant in real life. She started to help get the kids under control, so I could go and nurse the baby. Then Katy came in, crying, and she had a fever. I took her in my lap while I nursed the baby, not wanting her to feel jealous. Then the baby pulled away from my breast and threw up all over Katy, who really started to howl and bawl. (I woke up with my heart pounding, thinking, oh God, that's the way it's going to be!)

Blanche decided not to breastfeed her newborn boy "to avoid Katy's being jealous." She also commented, "This was a hard decision and I still feel guilty about it, as I'd really wanted to nurse. But Katy has been very sick all the time I've been in the hospital, so I think her needs are important too." To compensate for not nursing, Blanche allowed her milk to come in, and then expressed and froze it so that for the first six months, the new baby got the nutritional advantages of breast milk. Also, Blanche, her husband, and the part-time caretaker were careful to hold the baby when he was bottle-fed, giving him the bonding he needed.

Coping with Fears of Being an Inadequate Parent

Just as with the other six major fears of pregnancy, the first step in coping with this type of anxiety is to become aware of it. Often, pregnant women avoid facing the possibility that they might not be able to manage motherhood, yet their dreams and their diary records reveal these concerns. Until you admit this source of tension and nightmares, you won't achieve the deep relaxation needed both now and during the delivery. Your dream diary also should provide clues to the nature of other unexpressed anxieties.

WHAT OTHER COUPLES DO

Once you've analyzed your dreams and found they represent fears about your parental abilities, find out what others do in similar circumstances. If you're in the first or second trimester, try to attend at least a few early pregnancy classes. Check your yellow pages, ask your doctor, and call local hospitals to find such classes or lectures in your vicinity. These are usually free or quite inexpensive.

Begin attending childbirth preparation classes during your third trimester and make friends with other expectant couples. Remember that these courses are designed to help you. Don't be shy about asking the instructor any question, no matter how inexperienced it may make you appear. You will probably be surprised to find that most of the participants share your concerns.

In *Pregnancy Nine to Five,* Susan S. Stautberg, a mother and successful career woman, advocates careful planning in order to look and feel your best while working pregnant. She comments that some new mothers adapt to returning to work quite easily, while others need more time to adjust. When devising your schedule, try getting your employer to agree to an alternate, later date in case you require more time to make this transition.

AFFIRMATIONS AND CREATIVE DAYDREAMS

If you and your partner have done your best to prepare for parenthood but continue to fear inadequacy, practice deep relaxation and then repeat the affirmations designed to strengthen your self-confidence. (A number of these appear in the Appendix.)

In addition to the daily repetition of these affirmations (or others you may wish to compose in your own words), the integration of a creative daydream is an effective method for reducing anxiety. For example, after dreaming of being "all thumbs," Amelia used the same symbols to build a more positive self-image. First, she reversed the underlying, negative thought of the dream into the positive statement: "My love for my baby will give me steady hands and a sure, gentle touch." Amelia then relaxed deeply and created this beautiful daydream:

> I am in our garden with our new baby. I've dressed him in a little yellow tee-shirt and his diapers. I sit in a lawn chair and gently spread sunblock lotion on his exposed, tender skin. My touch is sure and delicate. He kicks and coos with pleasure. Then I put him down on a blanket in the shade while I weed the vegetables. I pull the weeds with no problem. My hands are strong and steady. Then the baby starts to cry. I take a deep breath and calmly wash my hands under the hose. It won't hurt him to cry for a few moments. Drying my hands on a cloth, I then pick up my baby and rock him, crooning soothing sounds. He's wet so I put him on the blanket and change his diaper. My hands are steady and sure. I feel confident and think what a calm, loving mother I am.

Some new parents have told me that these affirmations and creative daydreams have helped them even more after the baby was born. Amelia, for instance, said she found the above daydream most comforting during the first weeks after delivery. When her baby reached the ripe old age of three months, she commented, "Now I can't believe I went through all that agony and doubt about myself as a mother. It seems to me I was *born* being a mother. It just comes naturally. Oh, I made a few mistakes, like putting his clothes on backwards, and the first disposable diapers we bought were much too big. But nothing really serious happened. If I didn't have my journal to look back on, I wouldn't even remember how worried I was."

If your own dreams reflect this type of anxiety, reduce the

source of the tension now. Remember that any continuing worry can undermine your health and that of your baby. While parenthood is never easy—and can be even more difficult with a job or other children—millions of women have found ways to overcome these problems. Almost all of the mothers I have interviewed said that planning ahead and gaining their partners' support and cooperation were the most important factors in their ultimate success.

CHAPTER 11

❖

Dreams of Loss of
Your Mate

Do your dreams depict your partner as being sexually or romantically involved with another woman? Are you having nightmares that something terrible has happened to your husband? Such dreams appear quite natural, since pregnancy makes you feel more dependent on your mate. It's only normal to worry that something might happen to him.

Such dreams have worried many pregnant women for generations. The difference nowadays is that modern women often have difficulties "surrendering" to these dependency feelings. Since the 1970s and the women's movement, we've been taught to cherish our independence and equality. Thus, the expectant mother's naturally growing dependency may throw her into conflict. The result is that many contemporary women repress their personal and temporary needs, as well as their fears that they may lose their partners. Dreams often reflect this tension.

Dreams of Infidelity

Doris, a 32-year-old magazine editor, had this dream in her seventh month:

> In this dream I go to my old office to pick up a sweater I forgot. When I walk in, there is Karen, the woman who took over when I went on maternity leave, lying on top of my desk making out with a man. I say, "Oh, excuse me!" and start to walk out when the man looks up and I see it is my husband, Charles. I am stunned! (I woke up very upset, crying and angry at Charles. He told me it was only a dream and that he loves only me, but I can't help wondering.)

Dreams like Doris's are quite common during pregnancy. In almost every instance they stem from the dreamer's low self-esteem, due to both a denial of dependency needs and a desire to meet unrealistic body-image standards. The expectant mother also believes that as her waistline expands, she's no longer sexually desirable.

Doris made a confession in class: she had had sexual fantasies and dreams about herself with a former lover; these dreams were no more true of her waking behavior than was her dream that Charles was having an affair. Doris did the right thing by telling her husband about the nightmare. By getting this fear out in the open, she got the reassurances she needed.

Many of my students were comforted by a different interpretation of the "other woman": that this "third party" in dreams may represent the new baby.

For example, Sophia, a 33-year-old public relations agency manager, had this dream in her fourth month:

> I get home from work and Glen is sitting on the sofa with a young woman maybe seventeen or eighteen. He has his arm around her and is kissing the back of her neck. He sees me and says, "Oh, now our Mommy is home, darling.

Come over here, Sophia" and he beckons me over. I'm furious. "How dare you kiss another woman in our house!" I scream. "But she's so cute," he says. "Just look at her. Those big blue eyes look just like yours." (Then I woke up feeling both angry, hurt, and puzzled.)

When we discussed Sophia's nightmare in our couple's dream study group, Glen said, "Maybe the girl really did look like you, Sophia. Do you remember?" After some thought, Sophia said, "Yes, I guess she did look like a younger version of me." It was then that the other members helped Sophia to see that the young woman in her dream might have been her unborn child.

If such an interpretation of your own dreams makes sense, then by all means make use of it: your dreaming self may be telling you to share your love with the unborn child.

However, most women with infidelity dreams usually don't interpret the "other woman" as a symbol of the baby. Thirty-year-old Melinda, a court stenographer and wife of an airline test pilot I'll call Bob, also dreamed about her partner's affair. These dreams were so vividly realistic that Melinda was half-convinced they might be true.

When I examined the pattern of Melinda's dreams, though, another source of anxiety emerged. Here is a typical dream from her diary during the second trimester:

> Dreamed I parked at the shopping center and saw a pickup truck that looked like Bob's. But he was supposed to be at the airfield on the other side of town. When I went into K-Mart, I thought I saw him but when the man turned around, it wasn't Bob. Did my shopping and then up at the check-out there was some kind of commotion. The woman in front of me in line said a man had jumped over the counter and was raping the check-out girl. There were sirens and the police came. They pulled a man out and handcuffed him. From the back it looked like Bob and I thought, no, it must be that other guy I saw before. But then he turned to face me and it really was Bob! He looked very angry, not ashamed of anything. I was shocked.

(Woke up and felt jealous all day, feeling sure Bob was having an affair.)

At first reading, the above dream merely seemed to place Melinda in that group of women who feared becoming less attractive to their partners. However, that was before we examined all of Melinda's dream patterns.

Dreams of Your Partner's Illness or Death

We discovered that in her third trimester, Melinda had this nightmare:

> I was at my mother's house. . . . We heard this roaring outside . . . ran out to see several planes overhead. They were smoking, on fire, and about to crash. Several men bailed out, but their chutes didn't open. . . . I ran to try to help. Meanwhile one plane crashed into Mom's house and it caught fire. I could hear Mom screaming that my cat was burning up alive, but I kept on running. The trees where the men had fallen were burning too. I tried to drag one flyer out, but he was all tangled up in his burning chute. I saw that he was Bob and I began to cry. There was nothing I could do.

When viewed along with earlier dreams of Bob's infidelity, we can see a pattern indicating Melinda's intense fear of losing her mate. Either he will be unfaithful, or be taken away by force, or will perish in some horrible disaster such as a plane crash or fire. By noticing all the dream symbols, we can surmise that Melinda suffered from many anxieties as her due date approached. For instance, she seemed to have some unresolved conflicts with her mother. Further, if disaster should strike, she worried that she'd lose her unborn child (symbolized by the cat).

In her interview, Melinda told me her feelings see-sawed between depending on Bob and allowing him to take care of her, and then resenting the fact that she needed him more as her pregnancy progressed. "I feel so helpless sometimes," she commented. "Little things I used to do for myself, I just can't manage anymore. Sometimes I hate it that I have to ask Bob, even when I know he likes to take care of me." As our discussion continued, Melinda confided her worst fear: that something might happen to Bob and he wouldn't be there for her during the delivery.

Unwed Mothers' Dreams

Melinda and Bob had been living together for three years before they decided to have a child. Both their parents were pressuring them to get married. Her mother warned her repeatedly that unless they wed, Melinda would have no legal rights to ask for child support if Bob left her. Nevertheless, Melinda and Bob stood by their own convictions and never married. After a somewhat long labor of sixteen hours, Melinda gave birth to a normal nine-pound, two-ounce baby boy.

Melinda's nightmares about losing Bob may have reflected insecurities she felt about not being legally married. A number of unwed expectant mothers share this unexpressed anxiety. Here are excerpts from some typical dreams:

> *Ida, 26-year-old boutique manager in her fourth month:* Dreamed Roger (my partner) was seen several times with a skinny blonde . . . my best friend saw them.

> *Loretta, 33-year-old veterinarian in her fifth month:* I am on my lunch hour and see Sean, my lover, up ahead, arm around a petite little woman, maybe a teenager.

> *Trish, 30-year-old saleswoman in her fourth month:* A nightmare when I was lost in a maze like a carnival funhouse . . . running, scared, being chased . . . saw Josh in the mirrors making love to a gorgeous woman I don't know.

All these dreams of infidelity appear to reflect a dwindling self-confidence in personal appearance and sex appeal. Note how the "other woman" in each dream was described—a skinny blonde, petite little woman, gorgeous—implying the expectant mother's envy or wish that she herself looked more attractive. Although their unmarried status might have added to their insecurity, these dreamers probably suffered more from low self-esteem.

Similar fears disturb women who boasted stable marriages before becoming pregnant. To date, no one has investigated a large enough sample of unwed pregnant women to conclude that lack of a marriage license increases anxiety about loss of the partner. It's more likely that this concern plagues most pregnant women, wed or not.

Coping with Fears of Loss of Your Mate

Do any of the negative thoughts in your dream diary reflect the fear that you will lose your mate? Instead of shrugging it off, repressing anxiety, or telling yourself "it's only a dream," now is the time to take a more aggressive approach—the direct one.

SHARING IT WITH HIM

Upon determining that you do, indeed, have these negative thoughts about losing your partner, tell him. You can explain to him that such fears are quite common during pregnancy and are probably unfounded but that you need his reassurances anyway. Let him know that you love him.

Simply getting your worries out in the open may be all you need do to dispel them. As Chapter 5 emphasizes, when you express your feelings—especially your fears—this acts as a kind of psychological safety valve, lessening anxiety. It will be even better if you experience a stronger catharsis by letting your partner hold you close while you cry.

If you're worried that your condition makes you less appealing sexually, take heart from the fact that most expectant fathers love their mates even more when they're pregnant. After all, your enlarging abdomen shows evidence of a man's potency and masculinity. Even liberated males are likely to take a secret, slightly macho pride in having conceived a child. Sound hard to believe? Here are a few quotes from expectant fathers:

Rudy, in Agnes' fifth month: Just seeing her walking toward me on the street turns me on!

Sean in Loretta's seventh month: Once we worked it out about her ridiculous jealousy, our sex life has been better than ever. I don't want to be a chauvinist, but sometimes I can't help feeling like beating my chest Tarzan-style and telling the world, "This is my woman!"

Carl, in Colleen's eighth month: Even though she doesn't feel comfortable now with intercourse, we still make love. Have to admit I like this maybe more than what we used to do!

Like Colleen and Carl, you may find intercourse uncomfortable or painful near the end of your pregnancy. Some women feel this way even sooner. In her fourth month, Ida complained, "One of the reasons I'm worried that Roger may have an affair is that our own sex life is almost nil. Sex just hurts me too much. Even though I start out feeling aroused, I tense up because I know it's going to hurt. Then Roger gets turned off."

To help Ida, I told her about the opinions of medical experts. According to the Columbia University College of Physicians and Surgeons' *Complete Guide to Pregnancy,* unless specific medical complications exist, sexual activity is generally not harmful throughout pregnancy. Most doctors do advise refraining from sex if the bag of waters has broken, to avoid possible infection or premature labor.

Various reports debate the expectant mother's interest in

sex. Some say that you're most easily aroused during the second trimester but that this dwindles in the third. Others hold that pregnant women's sex drives are naturally heightened throughout gestation. My own experience with hundreds of expectant mothers causes me to agree with the latter opinion; most of the women seemed aware of higher degrees of arousal than ever before, and this state continued throughout their pregnancies.

Your own and your partner's preferences nevertheless remain the only important considerations. If you are avoiding sex out of fear, rid yourself of this needless anxiety. Your doctor or midwife will tell you that intercourse cannot harm the fetus, except under special circumstances.

If intercourse is painful or uncomfortable, especially in the missionary position (man on top), experiment with other positions. You may want to switch places. This will give you better control of the depth of penetration. Or, a side-by-side or rear-entry position, with you on hands and knees, could be more comfortable. Many couples find that experimenting in a playful way adds more excitement to their sex life than they've ever had before.

In your last trimester, honestly examine your feelings about sexual activity. Do you avoid it because you think your enlarged breasts and abdomen are unsightly? Your partner probably feels just the opposite. Ask him. If he admits that intercourse doesn't appeal to him right now, you can still enjoy oral sex and massaging each other to orgasm.

If you are fatigued and worried, sex may be the last thing on your mind. Yet, the emotional and physical release of orgasm can lift your spirits and make you more energetic. Try changing the time of day you and your partner enjoy intimacy. Perhaps you'll cherish it more in the mornings before the strain of the waking hours has tired you. On weekends or whenever you're together during the day, you might feel more like cuddling and embracing after you've had an afternoon nap.

CREATING DAYDREAMS AND AFFIRMATIONS

If you have shared your fears with your partner and made efforts to improve the quality of your intimacy with him but still find your dreams reflecting needless fear, create a positive daydream.

Doris, whose dream of catching her husband Charles "making out" with Karen was quoted at the beginning of this chapter, composed the following positive daydream to help her dispel worries that her husband might be unfaithful:

> I go to my old office to pick up a sweater I forgot. Karen, who took my place, is sitting at my desk. Charles is there, too. Together, they're looking through the desk drawers. I say, "Oh, excuse me!" and start to walk out. But Charles calls me back. He says, "I came by to get that sweater you forgot, honey. Karen was just helping me look for it. Where'd you leave it, anyway?" He puts his arm around me and says to Karen, "Doesn't she look fabulous?" and I can tell he's really proud of me. Karen says, "Oh yes. You look positively radiant, Doris. And I have some good news, too." Then Karen tells us she just found she is pregnant. She says, "Maybe you'll take my place when I go on leave, Doris," and we all laugh. We find my sweater and Charles helps me put it on. I say that as long as we're both here, maybe we should go out to dinner. We tell Karen good-bye and leave. Then Charles says, "After dinner, honey, let's go home and make love. You really turn me on these days!"

Doris reported to my Relaxation in Pregnancy class that she persuaded Charles to help her integrate this daydream by reading it to her. "After that," she told us, "Charles really proved to me that I really do still turn him on."

Another way to rid yourself of the unrealistic fear of losing your mate is to practice repeating affirmations that your partner loves and supports you. First, find a quiet time and place, breathe deeply, and follow instructions for Progressive Relaxation given in Chapter 3. Then repeat to yourself (or have your partner read) either your own affirmations or those in the Appendix.

If you continue to have nightmares after practicing deep relaxation, creating positive daydreams, sharing fears with your partner, and repeating affirmations that he loves you and supports you, an incubated dream may help. Melissa, a student in one of my Early Pregnancy classes, tried this technique. First, she used the Autogenic Training method described in Chapter 3 to relax deeply. Melissa opted for this technique rather than Progressive Relaxation because her anxieties were preventing her from going to sleep easily. Then, as she drifted off, she repeated to herself, "I will dream that Gary shows me how much he loves me." The next morning, Melissa recorded this unusual dream:

I dreamed I was up in the tree house my brothers and I used to play in as children. Only now I was pregnant and I couldn't get down. The ladder we used was broken. It was starting to rain with thunder and lightning in the distance. I felt very scared, afraid that lightning would hit the tree before I could get down. Then Gary started to climb the tree to help me. He had a tall metal ladder that extended high enough, but I still couldn't reach it. There was a big gap between the tree house platform and the ladder. He tried reaching out to grab me, but his arm just wasn't long enough. I was crying and sobbing and he kept telling me to calm down, that he'd get me out of there. The storm was getting worse and I don't think I've ever been so scared! Then I saw Gary taking out a long sharp-looking knife. I screamed, "What are you doing?" and he just smiled at me and began sawing away at the top of his right arm. It came right off, no blood or anything. Then with his left hand he held the cut-off arm and I grabbed its hand. That cut-off arm was alive! It pulled me over to the ladder and then, while I hung on, Gary somehow attached the arm to his body again. When I looked at it, you'd never know it had been amputated! It was amazing. Then he helped me down the ladder. On the ground, I was shivering and he took off his shirt and put it around me. (Then I woke up.)

When Melissa had shared her jealous feelings with Gary, he'd tried to reassure her by swearing he would do anything for her. "I'd cut off my right arm for you," he'd vowed. "I'd give you the shirt off my back." Melissa's dreaming self evidently took these declarations of love quite literally, presenting her with a dream depicting Gary doing exactly that! Melissa also thought this incubated dream was a precise illustration of another phrase she often used when confronted with a problem: "I'm really up a tree about this!"

Although some expectant fathers may, in fact, have affairs or fall victim to illness or accident, worrying about unlikely events will not prevent them from happening. It also may cause you to be unduly tense and unable to relax when labor begins. Release these tensions now, and let the love you both feel for each other and for your baby fill you with the peace and energy needed in the days to come.

CHAPTER 12

Dreams of a Difficult Delivery

Although women have worried about getting through childbirth for generations, today their concerns are more intense for a number of reasons. Many women have little or no emotional support, are older than the majority of mothers in previous eras, or are worried about the high incidence of C-sections. Others are anxious about the nudity and exposure the delivery will demand of them. Those with Superwoman Syndromes repress or deny their fears.

It's not surprising that many expectant mothers' delivery-related dreams are often nightmarish in quality and frequently have distinctive characteristics, such as

- Strenuous action depicting difficult trips or journeys
- Barriers the dreamer struggles to cross
- Tunnels, mazes, complicated underground structures
- Threatening characters: animals, robbers, intruders, monsters
- Environmental catastrophes: storms, fires, earthquakes
- Dramatic water symbols: ocean waves, choppy lakes, waterfalls
- Disasters: deaths, funerals, plagues, accidents

Dreams of Difficult Labor

For example, Eve, whose fears about losing her husband were described previously, recorded this "slightly scary" dream in her ninth month:

> I was at the ocean (it's a place I've never been but a place I dream about a lot). It's a rocky beach, the kind where you have to jump from rock to rock to get around. At this one spot there's a lot of big rocks, slanted with water rushing by them. I was hopping around. Came to a couple lying on this one rock. The man was really fat. Then I saw crocodiles in the water. They were really mean crocs! The man told me to watch out because they would take off my arm or leg. There were two men camped to one side of these rocks and they got over by swinging on a rope. I couldn't get by the fat man so I swung over on these guys' rope. Once I was on the other side, I began running fast.

Eve's dream clearly reflects worries about her rapidly approaching delivery. Indeed, it contains many of the characteristics described above—the difficult journey, barriers, threatening animals, and dramatic water symbols.

With your new interpretation skills, you already may have spotted diverse childbirth symbols in Eve's dream. The ocean represents the amniotic waters surrounding the fetus, as well as their breach and the ensuing labor contractions; the crocodiles symbolize both the fetus and the dangers Eve associated with the delivery; the rope stands for the umbilical cord; the fat man depicts Eve's self-image; and finally, the difficult struggle to get beyond the dangerous waters and her fast running at the end predict the outcome of her labor. In fact, Eve described her eight and one-half-hour delivery as being "very hard and fast," perhaps confirming an advanced knowledge of her body and the birth process.

Furthermore, although she reported being slightly frightened, she took positive action to get herself out of a dangerous situation. Eve repeatedly displayed this trait, even in her most scary nightmares. She also was different from most of my other research participants in that she openly admitted her fears.

The following are excerpts from other nightmares about difficult labors. Notice that all these dreamers appeared assertive:

> *Kitty, 22-year-old saleswoman:* Had to climb over this high wall . . . a panther waited at the top. . . . I hit him with my purse and got over the edge.

> *Olympia, 29-year-old ballet teacher:* Surfing in an ocean storm . . . fell off and saw a fierce looking white shark . . . banged it with the board . . . yelled for help.

> *Faye, 32-year-old advertising copywriter:* The basement of our house had changed into many rooms. All were flooded with bloody-looking water teeming with huge, mean rats . . . got lost down there . . . found a shovel and beat the rats away.

These typical nightmares contain many symbols of arduous labors and deliveries: strenuous or difficult journeys (Kitty's climb, Olympia's surfing); barriers (Kitty's high wall); underground structures (Faye's mazelike basement); threatening animals (Kitty's panther, Olympia's white shark, Faye's huge rats); environmental threats (Olympia's storm, Faye's flood); and dramatic waters (Olympia's stormy ocean, Faye's bloody-looking water). Each of these dreamers managed to be assertive in the face of danger; all three had labor under ten hours.

Conversely, Angela remained naturally demure and nonassertive. When she joined my research project, Angela was 32 years old, expecting her second child, and working part-time as a beautician. Since her husband refused to enroll in Lamaze classes with her, she attended the classes alone.

Angela told me that it didn't bother her that her husband wouldn't be her coach during delivery. "Larry works real hard," she explained, "And his baby-sitting with our four-year-old daughter saves money when I go to the classes." My intuition was that Angela did feel hurt by her husband's lack of total support. This seemed to be borne out by the following dream, reported near the end of Angela's second trimester:

> Larry and I were coming home from shopping, driving in the Toyota and going over the First Street overpass. When we stopped at the light, I looked down at our daughter in the back seat. She was asleep. When we turned left, the first thing I saw on the right was a huge barn burning. The flames were all on top of the barn. It was burning down fast. I thought at the time that there were probably a lot of little animals in there—and cows, being burned alive. There were people around, just watching. Nobody seemed excited or anything; they calmly walked by. By then we pulled up in our own driveway like we normally do. I remember feeling guilty. I wanted to do something, but it was too late. I woke up thinking, "Nobody cares, nobody cares at all!"

When we discussed this dream, Angela admitted feeling that "nobody cares" probably related to her husband's attitude. We thought the burning barn might symbolize her pregnancy, since she had undergone a C-section with her first child and feared another. Angela hoped for a vaginal birth, the motivating force behind her attendance at Lamaze classes. As it turned out, she did have a C-section again, after a lengthy labor.

Nearly all the dreams Angela reported were unpleasant and left her with vague feelings of guilt, frustration, or annoyance. It's possible that she might have had a shorter labor—and possibly a vaginal delivery—had she been taught to recognize the stress symptoms and anxiety revealed by her dreams.

However, no amount of dream study or relaxation can change certain physical conditions, such as a pelvis too small for your baby to get through. In these cases, deep relaxation before and during delivery may facilitate childbirth and help in recovery.

Coping with Fears of the Delivery

If you fear getting through the delivery, use the same techniques described for coping with other sources of anxiety. These include gathering information, incubating dreams, creating and integrating positive daydreams, and practicing affirmations designed especially to eliminate this specific concern.

Some fears about delivery are perfectly natural and nominal, but the modern feminine drive to be and do all things perfectly often traps today's pregnant women. Many expectant mothers feel that if they harbor any worries—especially about the "elemental" task of bearing a child—they somehow will be branded as incompetent or even traitors to their sex.

This is simply not true. Since ancient times, childbearing has inspired awe and even reverence. It also has evoked entire religions, cults, rituals, and branches of medicine. However, no pregnant woman was ever expected to bring forth a new life at least twice the size of her abdomen without fear, strain, discomfort, and a certain amount of pain. You do not have to do this perfectly or superhumanly, nor should you be ashamed if the prospect frightens you.

DEEP RELAXATION

No one claims that working with dreams or other states of consciousness will guarantee a painless, shorter delivery. However, I can promise that ridding yourself of unnecessary fears, routinely practicing relaxation techniques, and paying attention to both your sleeping and waking states will make childbirth easier, regardless of any complications that may arise.

Delivery comes more rapidly to those with a calm attitude. Also, if you're not tensing against each contraction, the pain will be greatly diminished and perhaps absent altogether.

Nervousness at the onset of labor, however, may cause the contractions to slow down or even stop. At this point, some physicians intervene with medications such as *pitocin,* a hormone that stimulates or increases contractions.

Bradley childbirth educator Carl Jones points out that contractions thus induced frequently prove quite painful and usually necessitates sedation of the mother. The fetal monitors also tend to show the baby in such distress that a C-section may have to be performed. Obviously, to avoid becoming trapped in this cycle, it's all important for you to take every possible measure to ensure that you'll be naturally relaxed when labor begins.

EMOTIONAL SUPPORT

To achieve a state of natural relaxation and serenity, emotional support from others—especially your partner—is all important. Numerous studies, including works of Dr. Grantley Dick-Read (*Childbirth Without Fear*) and Dr. Marshall Klaus and Dr. John Kennell (*Parent-Infant Bonding*) have established conclusively that pregnant women need someone else to share their feelings, fulfill their dependency needs, and encourage them to learn what to expect during the delivery.

According to almost every expert, the expectant father's support results in less difficult pregnancies and births. If your partner is reluctant to share childbirth preparation classes with you, news of these findings may persuade him.

Don't be shy about confiding your innermost fears. Eve, who dreamed of crossing the dangerous waters filled with crocodiles, may be an inspiration. "We started talking about our dreams and fantasies when we first began dating," she told me. "Now, we're best friends and we really believe all our feelings affect our health and our baby." Eve went on to say that her husband—a large, extremely virile man— surprised her with his interest in emotions, dreams, and other right-brain topics. Your own partner simply may be waiting for you to share your own concerns in order to safely confide his.

Emotional support and the single woman. If you are a single expectant mother, share the process with emotionally supportive friends. There's no reason to feel self-conscious about attending childbirth preparation classes with another woman (or a male, whether or not he's the father of your child). Numerous married women take a friend rather than their husbands, as do single mothers, for various reasons.

The essential point is to seek support from someone willing to make the commitment to attend the classes, practice with you at home, and be there throughout the delivery. If you cannot find such a person, talk to your childbirth instructor. He or she may know someone who would be delighted to act as your coach.

Dr. Marshall Klaus has initiated a program in some parts of the Midwest. Women who call themselves "doulas" lend support to expectant mothers during pregnancy and specialize as labor coaches. Also, instructors and midwives in training are frequently eager to gain the experience.

DELIVERIES WHEN YOU'RE OVER THIRTY

It's worth repeating that, unless diabetes or other serious health problems occur, the risk of childbirth remains extremely small for women under forty. Even forty-plus mothers now bear normal, healthy babies with comparative ease, provided they take appropriate precautions. Dr. Phyllis Mansfield, author of *Pregnancy for Older Women*, emphasizes the importance of finding an obstetrician who does not follow the century-old, traditional standards of advising child-birth only before mid-life. Such a physician should realize that women are generally in better health today than ever before. He or she also will understand the latest medical technology and not automatically tell you that you're at risk simply because of your age.

SURGICAL PROCEDURES

If you're worried about the rapid rise in C-sections recently, find out your doctor's and the hospital's policy about cesareans. Remember that one of the reasons for this increase is that modern technology now provides physicians with more information as the labor proceeds. Therefore, C-sections frequently help obstetricians intervene to prevent serious birth defects.

In your childbirth preparation classes, you will receive information about this surgical procedure and what you can expect if you must undergo it. Sometimes, merely identifying a specific worry may be all that's needed to dispel it.

Unlike most of the women I've studied, Beverly openly expressed her fears. In fact, she complained to all who would listen that she was miserable and hated being pregnant. "Childbirth is not a beautiful experience!" she emphatically stated. Yet Beverly's actual delivery was comparatively easy. She may have achieved a kind of catharsis by constantly releasing her tensions.

One aspect of delivery that particularly bothered Beverly was the possibility of undergoing an episiotomy, the incision of the birth opening to avoid tissue rupture as the baby emerges. After a slide presentation depicting this procedure, Beverly commented that it was "totally uncalled for" and showed "ugly, graphic pictures." She also believed it caused the dream she had that night:

> I keep seeing the worst pictures in the presentation (scissors, blood, ugly angles, and all). The doctor comes into

the labor room and I am screaming and thrashing about. He tells me that there isn't a chance he can find time to give me an epidural (which, in my "real life" he has promised me I can have)! He leaves me to have the baby alone. I am screaming, but he won't come back. (I woke up and cried hysterically for an hour and a half. It was terrible!)

As it happened, Beverly did not need an episiotomy. Her obstetrician was opposed to performing this incision except in emergencies. Furthermore she learned from her Bradley instructors perineal massage, a technique that probably enabled her birth canal to stretch without tearing during delivery.

This is not a recommendation to follow Beverly's example by complaining about every bit of discomfort occurring throughout your pregnancy. Rather, this true anecdote emphasizes that expression and the sharing of fears eliminate stress. A more moderate style than Beverly's would no doubt serve most women better in their efforts to achieve peace of mind.

ASSERTIVENESS AND LABOR DURATION

The women I've studied who were able to be even mildly assertive in scary dreams consistently experienced shorter labor than did those who were continually victimized. Sometimes this assertiveness is dramatic or violent, such as Kitty's knocking the threatening dream panther off the wall or Olympia's banging the attacking shark with her surfboard. At other times the dreamer merely protects herself by talking back to unfriendly characters or calling for help.

Anna, a 30-year-old secretarial services manager, had many nightmares reflecting concern about the delivery process. Early in her pregnancy, she appeared helpless, at the mercy of a variety of environmental dangers and attacking strangers.

Anna's fears decreased as she informed herself about the

minimal risks of delivery by attending childbirth preparation classes. Then, with the due date approaching, her
dreams began to be more assertive. She submitted this report
a week before her baby was born:

> Dreamed my contractions started coming fast. My hus-
> band was out of town. It was 3:30 A.M. and the lights
> wouldn't go on. I couldn't see my calendar and couldn't
> remember my due date. So I called my doctor and he came
> for me in a beat-up old Chevy. I had the baby on the way
> to the hospital without any help from the doctor. We were
> frantically looking for some string to tie the cord. Every-
> thing in the car was a mess, blood all over the seats. But
> the baby was calm and very peaceful. The car was rushing
> along a bumpy road the whole time! I felt really proud that
> I was strong enough to do it on my own and woke up
> feeling very happy.

The dream quoted above began with numerous small things
going wrong—no lights, husband away, loss of memory, and
so on. Then Anna gets real support from her doctor, delivers
without his help, and they work as a team after the baby is
born. By merely paying attention to the patterns of her
dreams, Anna experienced a type of spontaneous healing.
She reported feeling calm and confident as her labor began.

If you find yourself being victimized in any of your nightmares, they may be showing you that you are too passive or
submissive in some areas, such as your relationships with
your partner, friends, and relatives. Perhaps you need to
express your true feelings more openly, without so much
concern for others' thoughts. As you become more assertive
in your waking life, you probably will begin to defend yourself from nightmarish threats—or at least ask for assistance
from a friendly dream character.

DREAM INCUBATION

If you're trying to be more assertive during your waking life
but are still being victimized in your nightmares, dream
incubation sometimes can help. Review Chapter 7 for direc-

tions on choosing a dream topic. Then, as you drift off to sleep, repeat to yourself over and over, "I will be assertive in my dreams tonight" or "I will defend myself against any threats in my dreams tonight."

Heather, a 28-year-old telephone operator, was upset about constantly being threatened or physically attacked in her nightmares. When two weeks past her due date, she incubated this dream:

> Dreamed I was getting obscene phone calls at work. This one guy whose voice sounded like my doctor's kept ringing me and cursing me because he was getting the wrong number. I couldn't figure out how he was able to get me as his operator each time. First I told my supervisor but she just said, "Don't take it personally," which didn't help me at all because he kept on calling me. Then, instead of being polite the way we're taught by the company, I really told him off in spades! The supe came over and said, "You could be fired for this," and I told her where she could go, too! Then, the ceiling of the switchboard room suddenly caved in and a big flood of water came pouring down all over us. The other girls all started screaming and running out. I stayed put, got the maintenance department on the line and also the emergency crew. Then I left the room and everyone was cheering me. I was the hero of the day. (Then I woke up, soaking because my waters had broken. I felt so happy because this meant my labor had finally started. Also, I felt really good about that dream.)

Heather thought the annoying caller, with a voice reminding her of her doctor, symbolized delayed labor. "The day before I incubated this dream," she told us, "I'd been for a check-up and my doctor was questioning me about the date of my last period. I got the idea he suspected I'd been careless or had lied about it, making his calculations of my due date come out wrong, and that hurt my feelings." Heather thought this was the reason her dream supervisor advised her not to take it personally. She also explained that her doctor appeared unusually busy that day and that her appointment had not been scheduled. "He was probably just a little stressed and I was just too sensitive," she concluded.

Even before the ceiling caved in and her office flooded, Heather had taken assertive action by talking back to both the nasty caller and her supervisor, who she thought also symbolized her doctor. "I should have told him he hurt my feelings," she commented, "and I did . . . when we met a few hours later at the hospital. Then he apologized and we laughed about it."

Heather's labor was a brief four hours. Despite a pregnancy marred by very frequent nightmares of victimization, it's quite probable that her incubated, assertive dream helped Heather let go of some concerns troubling her at a very deep level of consciousness. She seemed to be almost totally relaxed during her labor and delivery and gave birth to a healthy, six-pound, three-ounce girl, with no complications.

CREATIVE DAYDREAMS

As you get closer to your own due date, you may find yourself having vivid, realistic dreams about your delivery. If these dreams reflect fear of unusual pain or unexpected complications, you can reverse your negative thought into a positive statement, creating a daydream designed to help you eliminate anxiety.

For example, Glenda worried about being unable to endure the pain of labor. "I don't want to have to ask for drugs," she told us, "because I know that's not good for the baby. But I don't know how I'll be able to stand it. I'm a real sissy when it comes to the least little bit of pain."

Three experienced moms provided Glenda with their personal stories. A homemaker, Fern had insisted on being given sedation during an earlier childbirth.

> It was at the end of the first stage of my labor. The contractions were suddenly coming hard and fast and it frightened me. When I tensed up in fear, the contrac-

tions were excruciating. So I started yelling for the nurse or my doctor to give me some painkillers. Well, everyone was bustling around, giving orders, whispering, and that scared me even more. My husband didn't know what was happening. He was just numb with fear and was holding my hand so tight, that hurt too. I started to try to breathe slowly and deeply, and then the pain began to fade. Anyhow, by the time they got to me with a shot of Demerol, I didn't even want it any more. But the nurse who gave it to me insisted, saying it was "doctor's orders." The result was that my baby was born about half an hour later and I couldn't even feel it. What a disappointment!

Edith, another woman with older children, nodded in agreement as we listened to Fern's story. "The same thing happened to me," she told us. "But we had a midwife who just took over from my husband and began rubbing my back, and helped me get into another position—on all fours, as I recall. Anyhow, she was talking to us all the time, telling us that this was just what she called the bridge between stage one and stage two. And, just as she predicted, I didn't need any painkillers once stage two got really going. Then it was just pure excitement. We could see the baby! My husband held a mirror down there so I could actually see the baby's head. And, when it came time for me to push, it felt really good."

Nan, a recent arrival from Hawaii, described her first delivery experiences:

Everything was going fine for me, too, until I hit that same period between the stages. Just like Fern, I got scared and tensed up, making the pain worse. Then my husband Kirk asked me what it felt like. I said it was like being caught up in a huge ocean wave. Made me feel helpless and nauseous with fear. Kirk told me to grab his arm the next time it happened. Then I said, "Uh oh—here comes another one!" and grabbed onto him. He said, "Hang onto me, honey. Pretend we're body surfing just like we used to at home. Just let this wave carry us up and up. Take a deep breath and let it out real slow." Kirk talked to me that way in a calm, strong voice and I started doing what he told me. Closed my eyes and could actually feel this enormous wave lifting us up! Then, as the contraction faded, it seemed we just floated back down into a trough between waves. Soon Kirk got so he could sense when the next one was coming, and he talked me through it. I actually began to enjoy it! By the time our baby crowned, I was so relaxed it was amazing. I could feel everything, yet it was almost as if I was outside my body watching it happen.

Although Nan and Kirk discovered their method of "mental body surfing" without any training, an almost identical technique is taught in a course for childbirth instructors by Dr. Pamela Schrock of Chicago. Since so many pregnant women liken contractions to the ebb and flow of ocean waves, this imagery is often highly effective in promoting relaxation during labor.

Another helpful imagery is that of the petals of a flower opening. With our encouragement, Glenda used this metaphor to create her own daydream.

First, she reversed her negative thoughts into this positive statement: "When my labor begins, I'll be confident and relaxed." Next, using the experiences of her classmates, Glenda composed the following scene:

My contractions are coming about five minutes apart. They don't hurt. It's more like a pressure from inside. It's the baby's head pressing against my cervix from the inside. The muscles of my cervix and my uterus are rippling over my baby, massaging him and helping him press against the opening. As the contractions speed up, my cervix begins to open slowly. It spreads open like a flower gradually blooming. The petals slowly move outward with each contraction. Now, as I begin my transition into the second stage, I take long, deep breaths and exhale slowly. To ease the pressure, I try different positions. Lying on my side feels good, with my husband massaging my back. Now, as I enter the second stage, I can feel downward sensations. I know this is my baby entering the birth canal. I feel tremendously strong urges to bear down, to push. We put a mirror on the floor and I squat over it. I can see the baby's head. Gently, I reach inside and touch his head! Now, my husband reminds me to pant and not to push any more, to avoid tearing. The baby pushes his own way out and I lie down again. After the cord stops throbbing, the doctor lets my husband cut it with scissors. Then, they put the baby in my arms. He's beautiful and my husband and I say to him, "Welcome, welcome, little darling!"

By practicing this lovely daydream daily during the last weeks of her pregnancy, Glenda let go of her fears about the delivery. She gave birth to a healthy, nine-pound baby boy after eleven hours of labor. "It was a lot like my daydream," she reported. "There was some pain and what I did was to holler really loud. That somehow helped and it must have relaxed me, because then I was right into the second stage. During that time I was working hard—sweating, huffing, and puffing—but I don't remember it being painful. Just hard work. Then, finally when he crowned, it went easy and fast and in just a few minutes he was out. Now that's over, I can look back and see that my worries about it all were rather exaggerated."

As Glenda discovered, you must identify your fears if they become a source of stress in your life. Otherwise, they may sabotage your best efforts to remain relaxed during labor. Carefully review your dream records and pay attention to your daily entries of negative thoughts for indications of unconscious fears. Also, honestly remind yourself of your last reaction to descriptions of an actual childbirth. If your exposure was a film, did you look away, tune out, leave the room, or feel queasy? Did your eyes dart away?

COPING WITH MODESTY OR INHIBITIONS

Unless you are a health professional, a nudist, or a frequent viewer of pornography, it's unlikely you're accustomed to seeing adults' genitals. Therefore, you probably would react with surprise or even shock when suddenly confronted with explicit photos of a woman giving birth while others watch. In fact, much of your fear about the delivery may be due to these learned inhibitions.

Although modesty has its merits in society as a whole, it has no place in the delivery room. If all your concerns are compounded by embarrassment about your body, it's going to be almost impossible for you to relax during labor.

To overcome some of this unnecessary modesty, try looking at yourself naked, in privacy, in a full-length mirror. Play some romantic music and let yourself sway or dance to the beat. As you do this exercise, observe yourself from various angles. Try some labor positions and practice until you feel comfortable viewing your reflection.

Next, invite your partner to join you. While looking at yourselves in the mirror, stroke your abdomen and sing or talk to your baby. Lie down and spread your legs for a good view of your vagina. Imagine your body's gradual opening to allow your baby to emerge. If all this nudity, romantic music, looking, and touching causes arousal, so much the better!

The notion that pregnancy and childbirth are not sexual experiences defies all logic, since your condition came about because of intimacy. Anything safely stimulating your desires should be welcomed as another expression of your harmony and total love for each other. On the other hand, you may find intercourse uncomfortable, especially as you reach the last month or weeks of pregnancy.

If this should happen, you can still enjoy the intimacy of noncoital sex—touching and kissing, stroking and massaging each other. This probably will occur quite naturally if you practice the mirror technique for overcoming your body inhibitions and invite your partner to assist you.

After becoming familiar with the positions you'll take during labor, return to viewing or reading descriptions of childbirth. Note your reactions this time around. Continue practicing the mirror technique until you can confront these graphic descriptions without feeling squeamish. If you still are upset with anxieties about your delivery, try integrating some positive affirmations.

CHAPTER 13

❖

Dreams of Loss of Control

Having grown to take pride in their abilities to control difficult situations in the workplace and in their relationships with men, many expectant mothers feel bewildered and frightened when their emotions and bodies suddenly no longer respond as expected. Once again, the Superwoman Syndrome increases anxiety about this issue much more than it did several generations ago.

As a result, many expectant mothers have disturbing dreams with the following traits:

- Dramatic emotional outbursts by the dreamer
- Dreamer acting inappropriately aggressive or violent
- Dreamer depicted as clumsy, awkward, helpless
- Symbols of loss of control during the delivery

Mothers-to-be typically experience a fear of losing control during the first trimester and the first part of the second, when rapid hormonal changes take place. Once this condition stabilizes, usually by the fourth month, extreme mood swings fade and the emotions are more balanced and appropriate.

Early Pregnancy Dreams

The following excerpts from typical early pregnancy dreams illustrate this fear:

> *Brooke, 25-year-old social worker in her third month:* Visiting my welfare clients, I picked up a crying child and shook her . . . told the mother she should discipline her brat.

> *Dahlia, 20-year-old college student in her fourth month:* At the gym, some jocks bumped into me . . . it didn't hurt, but I started to cry. . . . One of them apologized and I hit him with a baseball bat.

> *Nita, 34-year-old homemaker in the second month of her third pregnancy:* In the backyard my kids were yelling like they do out there . . . went out and turned the hoses on them . . . they got sick . . . felt so ashamed.

All these dreamers were bothered by seemingly unexplainable, irrational mood swings. Even after they understood that rapid hormonal changes caused so many inappropriate emotions, they continued to worry.

Brooke thought the dream of losing her temper with her client's child symbolized a general emotional turmoil. "I'd had a rough day just before I had that dream," she said, "and one woman with her wild kids really got on my nerves at the office." Brooke continued, "Usually I'm very compassionate and understanding with these women because they're so stressed and desperate. But lately I have a hard time staying in control."

Dahlia said her dream of being so emotionally overwrought represented "the way I feel most of the time. Like crying half the time and then striking out at everyone the rest of the time." After discussing this dream, Dahlia could see that the jocks symbolized Wayne, her partner, and his friends—all football players. "I used to love having them hang around," she said, "but ever since I got pregnant, their rough housing and crude jokes either make me cry or get mad." Dahlia also thought her dream choice of a baseball bat to hit the offending jock was a metaphor for her frequent desire to "strike out" at everyone.

When we talked about Nita's dream, she told us the reason this one especially disturbed her: "I believe in helping my kids build their self-esteem," she explained. "I'd never hit them or hurt them to discipline. But right now it's all I can do sometimes to control myself. I'm afraid I might actually do something like I did in my dream."

Late Pregnancy Dreams

During the second trimester and the beginning of the third, most women forget about this fear. Then, as their bodies become heavier, it suddenly may reappear. For example, Peggy, a 27-year-old bookkeeper, reported this nightmare in her eighth month:

> I was in a parking lot outside Safeway. I couldn't lift the packages out of my cart because I was so pregnant. I wished I'd waited to shop when my husband Stan could be there to help. Then a very old man shuffled over and helped lift the bags. I felt very embarrassed. Then I got in my car and suddenly I was going down a hill and the brakes didn't work. The car headed out onto a waterfront pier. Just before crashing off the end of the pier, I woke up. (I was shaking and my heart was pounding and all I could think was that I can't swim. This was really a frightening nightmare.)

Peggy said she felt uncomfortably vulnerable and totally dependent on Stan for activities she was accustomed to doing herself. "This nightmare certainly gives you a good picture of the way I feel most of the time these days," she said. "Even a very old man can manage better than I can!"

When we talked about the car going out of control, Peggy agreed this symbolized perceptions of her approaching delivery. "I feel panicked whenever I think about labor," she confided. "Everything's going too fast and I'm not ready. I may just go totally bananas when it starts and not be able to control my breathing or do anything right."

As the delivery due date nears, many women fall victim to an emotional turmoil similar to Peggy's: several fears compounded at once. Frequent nightmares, as well as severe waking tension and stress, consequently result.

Candace, a 35-year-old mother of two who did not attend Lamaze classes or make any other preparations for this third delivery, told me about this dream. She had it a few days before her labor began:

> I'm in a grocery store. I come across a large loaf of bread molded in the shape of a hideous skull. It suddenly gets up and has a whole body. It's a monster on the loose! Then I am lying on a bed and someone comes in. This person is headless and is carrying the molded bread skull on a silver tray. I try to warn Bill, my husband, who is also on the bed, about the approaching headless bread monster. I take Bill's shotgun (which he actually got rid of, in real life, several months ago) and I try to shoot the monster, but I can't get the shotgun to work. (With the terrifying thought that I was about to be killed by this dreadful creature, I woke up, crying and shaking.)

Candace believed the headless bread monster represented a number of her fears. "It's been my experience that the most painful part of labor is when the baby's head comes out," she told me. "So I think the bread turning into a head stands for that." Candace also thought the monster symbolized the way she feared both she and her husband would react when labor started. "I'm afraid we're both going to lose our heads and we'll completely forget all we actually do know about delivery," she explained. "Last time, that happened even though we'd gone to Bradley classes."

Candace's labor lasted a little over 12 hours. "We didn't lose our heads," she told me. "Bill was very much in control and I couldn't have done it without him. I shouldn't have worried about the crowning—that turned out to be the best part of my delivery. It felt great to bear down, there was no pain by then, and I was very excited and happy because finally the end was in sight. But I do think if I hadn't been so worried before, my labor might have gone faster. I was just too nervous and tense from the beginning."

"Daymares"

When the fear of losing control continues to be unexpressed or repressed, the mind may find a release in what some women call "waking nightmares" or "daymares." These often occur during a hypnogogic state, that twilight of consciousness when one is drifting off to sleep or just rising. If a pregnant woman is unusually anxious, she may have such an experience instead of the more common daydream or fantasy.

Candace, who dreamed of the headless bread monster, reported upsetting daymares around the same time as her nightmare. This is the way she described it:

> This is not a dream, but I am putting it in my Dream Diary because it is just as weird as my real dreams are. It happened yesterday and I can't get it out of my mind. All day, I'd been jumpy and nervous. Kept imagining I heard someone, like a prowler, outside or even in the house. Around 4 P.M. I was reading and sort of dozing off. But I'm sure I was awake when this happened. I distinctly heard someone in the room, right behind me. I then saw a shadow of a man in front of me. Thinking Bill had come home early, I looked around. No one there. Began reading again. Heard the noises again and saw the shadow again. This time I sat very still, watching the shadow looming closer. Then it raised its arm and it seemed to have a long knife or sword in its hand. I started screaming and without looking back, I ran outside into the yard. I was still sitting there shaking and sweating when Bill got home. I even made him go inside and check before I'd agree to come in

to fix dinner. There was nobody there, no trace of a prowler or knife or anything. Thank God, Bill is now taking his vacation and should be home with me until my labor starts.

Candace was probably correct: had she been able to rid herself of her fears prior to labor, childbirth would have been easier. If your own dreams or waking states of consciousness reflect this type of anxiety, here are some steps you can take to reduce or eliminate it.

Coping with Fears of Loss of Control

Fear of losing control is less severe and devastating than the other sources of anxiety already discussed, because it usually subsides by your second trimester and won't return until the end of your pregnancy. Still, any anxiety—no matter how transient—should demand your attention and be dispelled as soon as possible.

MANAGING EARLY PREGNANCY UPSETS

It certainly is unpleasant to be afraid that at any moment you may make a fool of yourself by suddenly bursting into tears or lashing out at someone you respect or love. This predicament often becomes more distressing for expectant mothers who still work when it happens. Bianca, a 32-year-old advertising executive in her second month, complained, "I nearly lost my best account yesterday by acting very impatient and making some totally uncalled for remarks." To cope with such predicaments, it is necessary to discharge excess emotions safely, share them with your partner, and practice deep relaxation.

Emotional expression. While rapid hormonal changes trigger the mood swings of early pregnancy, the emotions that erupt actually may be valuable in releasing hidden tensions. Review Chapter 5, especially the section on expressing anger, and find a safe place to uncork the anxiety. Roll up those car windows and yell!

Sharing. Talk about your feelings with your partner or, if single, with a close friend, your minister, or a counselor. An embrace and perhaps the freedom to cry on someone's shoulder may help you release a lot of emotional pain.

You don't have to rationalize or explain your feelings. Just sob and moan until the tears come. A good cry probably will enable you to feel more stable and competent in facing the world, without worrying about inappropriate emotional reactions.

Deep relaxation. As with all types of anxiety, practice the methods of deep relaxation described in the first part of this book. Find a quiet, comfortable place free of distractions and take fifteen or twenty minutes just for yourself.

At the end of this relaxation period, be sure to tell yourself that you will emerge alert and refreshed. You also might add a phrase affirming your right to have all of these feelings and to express them in an appropriate manner.

This self-hypnosis usually helps curb sudden emotional outbursts without having to subdue the emotions involved. You will recognize your feelings but save their expression until you're in a safer place.

MANAGING THE FEAR OF LOSING CONTROL LATE IN PREGNANCY

Instead of allowing clumsiness and awkwardness to make you anxious, keep reminding yourself that this is nature's way of slowing you down. During these final weeks, your baby needs the nurturing you can best provide when relaxed and serene. Try to resign yourself to the idea that others will have to take over your usual chores or that you simply may have to reduce your load.

If your waking thoughts conjure up dread of losing control once labor starts, now is the time to dispel needless stress. You can achieve this through deep relaxation, dream incubation, integrating creative daydreams and affirmations, and getting in touch with your "birthing energy" and sharing it with your partner.

Deep relaxation. If you have been following my advice throughout this book, you already are adept at Progressive Relaxation and Autogenic Training. If not, please review Chapter 3 and give yourself the benefits of these easy enjoyable methods.

Taffy, a 28-year-old homemaker in her second pregnancy, told me: "My husband Phil and I look forward to our relaxing hour just the way we used to enjoy our cocktail hour. We put Junior in the tub and while he splashes, we retreat to the bedroom. It's a time just for us, when we can both unwind. After Phil leads me through the exercises, I do the same for him."

Whether you practice with your partner or alone, this regimen is vitally important during your third trimester. Progressive Relaxation helps you tap into the powers of your deeper consciousness to resolve any anxieties. Additionally, it trains your mind to control each set of muscles, a practice that facilitates labor. If experiencing severe stress or sleeping problems, use Autogenic Training as a special tool for relaxation and dream incubation.

Affirmations and dream incubation. Nightmares reflecting your fear of loss of control can be counteracted by some of the affirmations suggested in the Appendix. You also may use dream incubation to determine the meaning of frightening dream characters or elements. For instance, Martha, a 26-year-old secretary, reported this nightmare in her eighth month:

I had this terrible, scary dream. My husband and I were at home. There was an older woman there, but I don't

know who she was. A stranger was lurking outside. I felt
terrified. The woman opened the door and let the stranger
inside. He had a weapon! He and my husband began
arguing. I was totally scared, petrified! The scene went on
for quite awhile. The crazy, weird-looking stranger told
my husband he was going to hurt me somehow. This
really scared me as I was pregnant in the dream. (Before
anything happened, I woke up. I felt relieved it was over,
but it took me some time to feel safe and go back to sleep.)

To provide a better understanding of this nightmare, Martha
incubated it, following the instructions given in Chapter 7.
Here is the result:

In this dream I was at home again with my husband and
the unknown woman. This time, I see that the woman is
my mother. She is telling me that it is all right to let the
stranger inside, that he means no harm. I feel scared but
I agree. She opens the door and he comes in. I ask, "Who
are you? What do you want from me?" and he begins to
grow bigger until he's practically a giant about ten feet
tall! I feel more scared then ever, but my husband gets in
front of me and says, "I won't let you hurt her!" Then this
giant smiles and says, "I am your birth power. If you let
me stay here in your house, I'll help you bring the baby
outside. But if you fight me, then I'll have to hurt you."
And he holds the weapon up. We see it is a surgeon's
scalpel. My Mom says, "You see, I told you we had to let
him inside." (And I woke up.)

This incubated dream suggested to Martha that the house
represented her uterus. However, she did not associate the
intruding stranger with her unborn child. Rather, the giant
probably represented Martha's growing awareness of a new
type of energy presently invading her body.

Birthing energy. Many women in late pregnancy report
these feelings, although most cannot fully describe the sense
of being taken over or overwhelmed by some powerful
force. Rahina Baldwin and Terra Palmarini, midwives and

authors of *Pregnant Feelings* and *Special Delivery,* describe the onset of this birthing energy as sometimes occurring in late pregnancy and always presenting itself during active labor. One of the signs of birthing energy is what's been called the "nesting instinct," a strong urge in your last trimester to houseclean, redecorate, prepare a nursery, and perform other home-centered activities. Heaviness and fatigue may seem swept aside as you experience bursts of energy. Many women report similar feelings during labor, indicating the desire to make a pleasant environment for their babies.

Now is the time to consciously step aside, allowing this unexpected birthing energy to function without interference. Indulge yourself in extra rest and perhaps some type of recreation for which you haven't had time. Go to a movie or curl up with a good book. Let your partner pamper you, give in to your feelings of dependence, and share them with him.

In *Mind Over Labor,* Carl Jones speaks of birthing energy and labor as the opening of a window or a door. You may wish to create your own daydream with this analogy. Imagine your cervix slowly opening and widening until its aperture permits your infant's head to pass through. Your body wields the power for this event to take place. However, if you tense against the process, the door will be blocked, delaying your baby's entrance into the world.

Turning it over. When the fear of losing control accompanies other, more deep-rooted anxieties, body tension escalates. Such an accumulation of stress can make it all the more difficult for you to relax during labor. Many women find that they must focus with extra concentration in order to let go or turn the process over to those who want to provide support.

Moreover, even confident, relaxed couples often fear that with the onset of labor, they will lose control and forget the instructions they've learned so well. While it's undoubtedly an advantage to be skilled in the breathing techniques taught by childbirth educators, many parents-to-be also appear so determined to perform these methods perfectly that they lose sight of their purpose: relaxation during labor.

How your partner can help. One of the reasons childbirth instructors urge you to bring your partner or a friend with you to the delivery room is so that you will not have to worry about remembering the proper procedures for each stage of labor. Your "coach" reminds and encourages you. Begin to turn over control of these methods to your labor partner. He or she will not be alone, either—there's no law against your partner asking the midwife or doctor what to do next!

Expectant fathers who feel involved in their mates' pregnancy and the delivery experience higher self-esteem than those remaining aloof. So, when fears of becoming burdensome or overly dependent arise, rest assured that your needs make your partner believe he's a vital part of your mutual creation. As one of my students commented, "This is the one time I can be a child again. Soon, I'll have to take up my roles as worker, chief cook and bottle washer, and mother. Right now, I'm just enjoying the time we have to do little things together, like watching TV, going out to dinner or a movie, and especially just cuddling and talking. These are little things, but I know all this sharing is a time we'll never forget."

CHAPTER 14

Dreams of Financial Burdens

Unless fortunate enough to be among the very wealthy, you may be troubled by the prospect of the additional expenses the new baby will bring. The fear of insolvency frequently appears more pronounced in the mother-to-be than in her partner. Her paycheck is often as important to their livelihood as his, plus she worries about the additional stress soon to confront him.

Today's inflation exacerbates the whole problem. If you are worried about finances, rest assured that many pregnant women share your anxiety.

Media attention to the problems of the homeless also adds to your concern for your family's future. The increasing numbers of working mothers worry about their ability to continue on the job—or perhaps wish they could stop in order to be at home with their babies.

Some women needlessly ponder future expenses: private schools, orthodontists' bills, and college tuition. If you're prey to this type of anxiety, let go of it right away; you are undermining your health and that of your unborn child by fretting over issues you have no way of predicting or resolving.

Although I cannot offer you instant prosperity, I can share with you the experience of those who have learned to overcome their financial fears. But first, examine your dreams for clues that indicate this particular unexpressed anxiety. The most dominant themes and elements include

- Dreamer's or partner's career problems
- Dreamer's or partner's loss of job
- Partner portrayed either as irresponsible or overly stressed
- Dreamer (or family) in abject poverty, hungry, destitute
- Needy fetal symbols or children

Dreams of Career Problems

Sometimes dreams focusing on problems in the workplace may be reflecting other fears, such as your concern about balancing a career and motherhood or losing control. To identify and isolate the unexpressed, worrisome issue, review recent dreams that refer to your work or office settings. The method is explained in Chapter 6.

It's also possible for any symbol to contain several levels of meaning. Therefore, dreams depicting work-related problems may indicate your anxiety about parenthood, loss of control, or financial burdens. In fact, most pregnant women's dreams reveal a variety of symbols, with some representing two or more of the six major fears.

Mitzi is a 32-year-old stockbroker. After she and her husband Saul decided that he would stay at home with the baby and she'd return to work, Mitzi had this dream:

Saul was down in the basement of the house I grew up in. He was talking on the phone long-distance and I was furious . . . screaming obscenities at him and hitting him.

He just smiled in a patronizing way—which made me madder! I told him I was leaving and he could just forget about the baby . . . upstairs to pack, realized that all the clothes I was pulling out . . . weren't maternity clothes. I was very upset . . . back downstairs, feeling horrible, betrayed. . . . Saul had walked away . . . leaving the phone off the hook so we were still being charged. . . . My mood quickly shifted back to furious. Said really vicious things to Saul who just seemed not to care at all. (When I woke up, I was still mad.)

Mitzi's dream has many symbols common to pregnancy: places from the past (the house in which she grew up), architectural references to her uterus (the basement), and the mention of maternity clothes. Her anger at her husband surfaces in the comment that he "could just forget about the baby." This may have indicated both Mitzi's resentment that Saul was taking the approaching delivery more calmly than she did, as well as her doubts about the decision to leave the infant in his care. Notice how the dream portrayed Saul as irresponsible (leaving the phone off the hook).

Discussing her dream, Mitzi said, "I am beginning to feel really anxious about finances since I'll be the only paycheck once the baby is born." In another late pregnancy dream, these worries became more pronounced:

Dreamed the Dow went down to 400 (currently 2055). Made me very depressed but very calm . . . on the phone with a little boy client who owned three shares of Disney . . . half-listening, half-watching my machine . . . told the boy we were making history and I would get back to him . . . I started panicking, yelled to my secretary . . . she acted like I was overreacting. . . . She said an old friend of mine, Tom, wanted to talk to me, but he was behind a fence and couldn't come to my desk . . . something about him being a male stripper . . . told her I couldn't talk to him right now because of the market.

Again, Mitzi's dream contains pregnancy and childbirth symbols: the little boy client (a fetal sign) and the fence (a barrier representing labor) she must climb if she wanted to reach her friend Tom. At another level, Tom also may have depicted Saul, the man left "behind" to become a house-father. While this suggests Mitzi's concern about breaking with traditional male-female roles (note Tom's appearance as a male stripper), the major theme here is a market crash—clear evidence of the primary worry: finances. Such a disaster would have a direct, serious effect on the family.

As it turned out, the couple bore a healthy baby girl who is developing quite normally under her father's loving care. Mitzi says she spends plenty of "quality time" with her baby in the evenings and on weekends, while continuing to pursue her promising career.

Christine, a single, 34-year-old account executive, planned to work until her baby was born. When her doctor insisted that she start her maternity leave at the end of her eighth month, she commented: "This really upset me because I've been trying to save ahead in case I can't go back to work right away after the delivery. But my doctor says I need more rest to avoid complications later."

The first week of this imposed maternity leave, Christine was troubled by a series of nightmares. She described the following as "especially harrowing":

> Dreamed I was trying to phone my office to check on one of my biggest accounts. The phone cord had been cut so it didn't work. Then the extension in the kitchen wouldn't work either. I went to a pay phone and called the telephone company. They told me they'd cut off my service because they knew I wouldn't be able to pay the bills. I was furious and tried to tell them I'm on paid maternity leave. But the phone company person said, "That may be true, ma'am, but we have no guarantee you'll be able to return to work after your baby is born." I was so mad, I was shaking and dropped all the coins I had with me. They washed away in the water that was rushing through

the gutter next to the phone booth. Then I couldn't make the call to my office. Began to cry (and then woke up, still crying. This one upset me so, I couldn't get back to sleep and paced the floor until morning, when I could actually telephone the office).

Again, this dream contains typical pregnancy symbols: the cut phone cord (umbilical cord), the rushing water (labor and the waters breaking), and the gutter (birth canal). However, Christine's nightmare clearly demonstrates her fear of financial burdens and the possibility that she might lose her job while having her baby. In actuality, she stayed in contact with her office and clients by phone. Christine also returned to the same firm after the normal delivery of a healthy baby boy.

Dreams of Poverty

Career women are not alone in suffering from this anxiety. The dream diaries of nearly all expectant parents reflected the fear of poverty. Marion, a 25-year-old homemaker in her fourth month, recorded this nightmare:

After seeing a TV show about an ordinary, middle-class family that became homeless and had to go on welfare, I dreamed that I was a bag lady on the city streets. Maybe I'd already had my baby, because I wasn't pregnant in the dream. I was poking around in trash cans in an alley and felt very scared that someone I knew might come by and see me. Then I found a carton that was still warm and was full of fried chicken. This was a real treasure! I remember thinking I could feed my whole family with this. I put it in my shopping bag and started home. To get there I had to open a manhole and go down into the sewers under the sidewalk. It was horrible! The underground tunnels were full of damp and smelly puddles, and I thought I saw rats scurrying around in the dark. I kept striking matches trying to find my way. Then I dropped my bag and everything fell out and was ruined. I just stood there looking at the mess and cried and cried. (That's all I remember, thank goodness—because I think this awful nightmare got even worse before I finally woke up. In real life my husband and I are doing all right. He has a good job with a good future, so I don't have to work. Our budget will be pretty tight, though, with a new baby. So I guess it's only natural that we do worry a little.)

Note the childbirth references: the food (nurturing the un-born), the manhole and sewers (underground structures representing Marion's uterus and the labor to come), the damp, smelly puddles (again depicting labor), and the rats (typical early pregnancy fetal symbols). Apparently, Marion still felt ambivalent about her pregnancy and had rather foreboding perceptions about the way her delivery might be. Still, financial anxiety really proved to be the dominant theme.

Marion's viewing of a drama about a homeless family might have triggered this nightmare, but it evolved because of more deep-seated worries: in order to make ends meet, she thought she might have to begin working. Her strong desire to stay at home and nurse her baby thus prompted visions of being a destitute bag lady.

Dreams of Needy Babies and Children

This worry about financial burdens is also mirrored in dreams about impoverished babies and children. The following excerpts are typical:

Renatee, 20-year-old fashion designer's assistant, unmarried: My Mom gave birth to my baby, but she refused to keep it . . . told her I'd look for adoption agencies . . . got home from the shop and found a litter of starving kittens in my bed.

Dacia, 33-year-old movie theater manager: A documentary about starving African kids was showing . . . saw the audience was nearly all exactly like the children on the screen.

Carlynne, 27-year-old restaurant cashier: Every one of the customers had no money to pay . . . my boss threw a family
with hungry children into the street . . . I quit.

Renatee's dream reflected a number of her anxieties: fear of
a difficult delivery (her mother having her baby for her), fear
of being an inadequate parent (considering adoption of the
baby), and fear of financial burdens (the starving kittens).
This anxious mother-to-be had good reason to be so concerned. Although she and her live-in lover wanted the pregnancy, he had been in an auto accident and could no longer
work.

Renatee also experienced an agonizing conflict because
her parents refused to help them. "Mom and Dad told me
I brought this on myself," she explained, "so now I'd just
have to give up the baby for adoption. It's almost like they
want me and my baby to suffer, just to prove they're right,
that I should have gotten married. At least I do have medical
insurance or I'd probably have to go on welfare."

As it turned out, Renatee bore an eight-pound, four-
ounce boy after a C-section. Her employer gave her paid
maternity leave and even a promotion on her return to work.
By that time her partner had recovered sufficiently to take
care of the baby. Although unable to return to his job as a
construction foreman, he soon worked part-time in carpen-
try. "It's no bed of roses," Renatee said, "but still it's not as
bad as I'd feared. We feel we've come through the worst and
that from now on things will just get better."

Dacia's dream of the starving children and Carlynne's
nightmare of the hungry families give strong evidence of
their anxiety about finances and the expenses their new
babies might bring. "I may lose my job," Dacia said, "because our theater is being bought up by a large conglomer-
ate." It also developed during our discussion that this
mother-to-be had been actively involved in the Hunger Project for a number of years. She thought her dream indicated
both a concern with world issues and worries about her

personal livelihood. "It would be ironic," she commented, "if we had to ask for help now, after all the time and effort we've put into trying to stop starvation around the world." As it turned out, Dacia kept her job after giving birth to a healthy little girl.

Carlynne thought her nightmare reflected her relationship with her father, as well as her concern about finances. "I'm sure 'the boss' in my dream stands for Dad," she told us. "My boss is so tenderhearted he'd never turn away anyone who was hungry." Carlynne then explained that her father strongly disapproved of her marriage to someone of another faith and had not spoken to her for three years. She had never quite recovered emotionally from this rejection. However, when Carlynne's healthy baby boy was born, her father came to visit. "He was practically staggering under an armload of presents," she said, "and he cried and apologized. It was a wonderful reunion."

Coping with Fears of Financial Burdens

Once you recognize that financial worries are causing you anxiety, you have a number of options to dispel the fear:

- Sharing your anxiety with your partner or friends
- Getting temporary credit or loans
- Negotiating with creditors
- Learning about your rights to maternity leave
- Planning ahead
- Deep relaxation
- Integrating affirmations and creative daydreams

SHARING YOUR ANXIETY

Don't repress anxiety with the well-meant intention of sparing your partner from it. If you do, you run the risk of becoming overly stressed or tense so that your partner may worry about you anyway. More important, however, total communication provides the basis for a close and loving relationship. Simply discussing your concerns also clears up misunderstandings about how the two of you can meet additional expenses.

If you are a single expectant mother, it's equally important for you to confide in a close friend or relative. Expressing your fears is an effective way to release tension. Also, once you have articulated your worries, it will be easier to view them objectively and choose whatever action may be needed to prevent their return.

TEMPORARY CREDIT

Next, if you cannot meet your mounting bills, consider asking relatives and friends for temporary assistance. In their efforts to be independent, some couples keep financial problems to themselves, though their families and friends might be able to help.

Also, investigate the possibility of getting a loan or line of credit from your local bank. A relative or friend might be willing to co-sign, even if unable to personally advance you the money.

NEGOTIATING WITH CREDITORS

When I met my present husband, I was a divorced mother of two, struggling to make ends meet and frantically worrying about the ever-mounting bills. Coincidentally, this wonderful man was a C.P.A. and experienced financial advisor. At his suggestion, I telephoned all my creditors and made arrangements to pay small monthly sums until my debts were cleared.

Most creditors will cooperate by helping you set up a schedule of payments if you convince them you intend to honor your agreement. Once the stress of my financial situation eased, I was able to concentrate more on my job and soon got a promotion. Then I came out of the hovering black clouds haunting my dreams.

YOUR RIGHTS TO MATERNITY LEAVE

If you are a working mother and plan to continue your career after the baby comes, find out about your rights under the Federal Pregnancy Discrimination Act. Susan S. Stautberg, author of *Pregnancy Nine to Five,* and Jane Hughes Paulson, author of *Working Pregnant,* both explain that this law, passed in 1978, has a number of limitations. The Federal Pregnancy Discrimination Act makes it mandatory for companies with more than fifteen employees to provide disability insurance; pregnancy is covered as such. However, if you work for a smaller firm with no maternity compensation plan, this law may not help you.

Stautberg and Paulson both suggest that you immediately determine your company's sick leave, disability insurance, time-off, and paid maternity leave policies. Even if your firm carries insurance, you may not be covered unless you have met various eligibility requirements. Paulson offers one rule of thumb: you are entitled to the same coverage for pregnancy that other employees get for their "disabilities"—provided you meet the same requirements.

Benefits also vary from state to state. Firms with a strong social conscience may provide six weeks' paid maternity leave, while others only allow for the state's minimal insurance coverage—or none at all. If you work in a small company, you may be the first one to test these policies.

Certain minimum federal rights protect all employees. You cannot be fired or refused a job or promotion simply because you are pregnant. If you suspect discrimination or have other questions, call the local office of your state's unemployment department. The same government bureau can make suggestions about what to do if you need to stay at home for weeks or months without paid employee benefits. Some states have special insurance compensation programs for this situation.

PLANNING AHEAD

You and your partner also may be troubled about more distant financial burdens, such as your child's education. Even couples unable to put aside substantial savings usually can start a piggy bank account for the baby. Put aside a few dollars each week and allow them to earn interest. Meanwhile, keep in mind that scholarships and student loans probably will be available when your child is ready for college.

Still, some people make themselves needlessly anxious about financial burdens so far in the future that there's no way anyone could predict the outcome. Even generally optimistic women sometimes fall into this type of negativity when pregnant. Make an effort to put some humor in your life. Go to a comedy film, have lunch with a lighthearted friend, or indulge yourself in some small, frivolous treat.

DEEP RELAXATION

Whether you are a chronic worrier or actually have real cause for anxiety about finances, practicing deep relaxation remains so important to every client, every student, every pregnant woman I meet that I emphasize it in almost every chapter of this book. Chapter 3 contains simple directions for Progressive Relaxation and Autogenic Training, and I urge you to review them.

By putting aside all your anxieties for half an hour or so and letting go of all body tensions, you will do more than refresh yourself physically and emotionally: your deeper consciousness may lead you to new solutions.

DREAM INCUBATION

Try incubating a dream to clarify your interpretation of deep-seated financial worries. As you are drifting off to sleep, completely relaxed, tell yourself, "I will dream tonight about the (describe the puzzling dream element) and find out what it means." Then when you awaken, write down whatever you recall. If the answer does not come right away, put your diary aside. Usually a solution will occur to you at some later time.

You also can incubate a dream to rid yourself of negativity and needless anxiety. For example, Hedy, a 34-year-old homemaker and mother of a three- and a four-year-old, described herself as a "worry wart." After realizing in her eighth month that she herself was causing her fears about future expenses, Hedy told her dreaming self, "Tonight I will dream about ways I can stop worrying so much about money." This was her incubated dream:

> The scene reminded me of an illustration in one of my kids' story books. Perfect blue sky with fluffy clouds. Green hills in the distance. A sapphire blue river winding lazily through meadows of wild flowers. Hiked along a path. My girls scampered ahead, squealing, laughing. Then noticed they were wearing their new Easter outfits. Yelled, "Be careful! Don't mess up your new dresses—they cost a lot." But they paid no attention and went to the riverbank. Began wading, splashing. I was very pregnant, but I went as fast as I could to stop them. Too late, they were soaked and muddy. I started to cry, thinking how much I'd paid for those clothes, now ruined. Suddenly it started to storm and the river turned into an ocean. A ship came up as I dived in to save my kids. But the girls climbed up a ladder onto the ship to a woman holding out Easter baskets full of eggs. [They] sailed off [together]. I screamed, "You're kidnapping my children!" and then a big wave knocked me down. I was back on shore. Spitting out sand and water. Choking. To my amazement, there were both my girls, still in their

new outfits, sitting on the sand, just like nothing had happened. I was so glad to see them. Hugged them, took off their clothes. Told them to play and have fun, get as messy as they wanted. Then, it seemed so funny that I took all the new clothes and threw them back in the river (the ocean had changed back). I lay down on the bank. Breathed in the sun, and looked at the now peaceful scene. (Then I woke up, thinking it could be happy like that all the time.)

Hedy's incubated dream contains perhaps more pregnancy and birth symbols than a spontaneous one: water (at first a calm river, then a stormy ocean, reverting to a river again—similar to the ebb and flow of labor contractions); green hills, meadows, and flowers (representing growing things); her hike, running after the girls, the ship sailing away, being knocked down by waves, choking and spitting, and then lying back in contentment (all indicating a strenuous labor, delivery, and her recovery); and the basket of Easter eggs (fetal symbols).

Hedy said that this dream helped her realize that "right now is the most important. The Now is my priority!" Asked to clarify further, Hedy told us, "After this dream, for some reason my whole attitude changed. It was almost a religious experience and that's hard to explain. Somehow I just saw that worrying about material things doesn't do anything good for anyone in my family. In fact, it just drives away the people I love, if I'm always harping on taking care of things. Just like my girls sailed away in the dream. Now, just like in my dream, I've gotten a second chance so I've stopped bothering with money worries."

CREATIVE DAYDREAMS AND AFFIRMATIONS

Hedy also created a daydream as added insurance that she would cease fretting needlessly. By relaxing deeply and then having her husband Ralph read her the following, she integrated its message into her deeper consciousness:

We have had our baby and you and I have just gotten home. While you were at the hospital a lot of housework got piled up. Your mother is here to help and she's in the kitchen giving the girls their lunch. She hugs us and takes the baby so you can rest. In our bedroom, you take off your clothes and throw them in the hamper. "Sorry it's full," I say. "Oh, I don't care," you answer, "it's only clothes. They'll get done eventually." We both laugh and while you're putting on your nightgown I confess, "I didn't balance your checkbook or pay this month's bills, either. But now your Mom's here, I'll get right on it." You laugh again and say, "Plenty of time, darling. Let's cuddle before the baby's next feeding." And so we snuggle up. Then Mom brings the baby, with the girls skipping along, too, and we all sing a lullabye and hug one another as we watch the baby nurse.

"You may think this is a corny little scene," Hedy told our Relaxation in Pregnancy class, "but you wouldn't believe how hard it was for me to make it up, especially the part about the unbalanced checkbook and unpaid bills! It really did help me in my struggle to stop being a worry wart and give my attention to the love I feel from and can give to our baby and our family."

It's also time for you to focus your energies on providing a nourishing, loving environment for your baby. By all means, express your concerns about future financial problems, inform yourself of available resources, take reasonable action, and then let go of any needless worries regarding distant future. No matter what your income, you already are giving your child the most valuable gift: your love and dedication.

CHAPTER 15

Conclusion: Sweet Dreams

Although most of the dreams pregnant women recall are somewhat nightmarish or threatening, the moms-to-be who resolve their fears and learn to release anxiety start experiencing happier dreams as the due date nears. Regardless of the central theme or motif, most of the sweet dreams of late pregnancy usually possess some of these references:

- Water and other labor symbols
- Actual delivery scenes or symbolic deliveries
- Dreamer's partner, her mother, or both
- Healthy newborn infants
- Attractive fetal symbols

The Sweet Dreams of Late Pregnancy

Lydia, a 25-year-old tour guide, was typical of my students who learned to make a daily habit of deep relaxation. In the beginning of her ninth month, she had this dream:

> At the supermarket check-out counter, I bought several gallons of purified water and a five-dollar lottery ticket. The clerk gave me the ticket and then took it back. He put it on the computer and then told me, "You've won! Hold

on, I think you're a big winner!" Then hundreds of silver dollars began pouring out of the change-making machine. It was like hitting the jackpot in Vegas! The clerk gave me a shopping bag and I tried to catch the coins, which were piling up on the counter and spilling onto the floor. Other customers were picking them up and handing them to me. I stuffed my pockets and purse, and the money kept coming. It was incredible. The clerk said I'd won nine million dollars. People were cheering and a reporter was taking my picture. They asked me for a statement and I said, "All I did was pick the numbers that had to do with my pregnancy—the day I think I conceived and my due date." The reporter said, "Lady, if that's your due date, you'd better take care, because that's today's date." I was surprised because I thought it was a month away. Then the change machine burst open and there lying on all the silver dollars was a tiny baby boy. I picked him up and hugged him and everyone cheered. (I woke up, feeling blissfully happy.)

This dream clearly mirrors Lydia's pleasure in approaching the end of her pregnancy. "Once I learned how to relax— and I mean totally, not just on the surface—everything seemed so easy," she explained. "I sort of floated through the last couple of months. The things that used to worry me began to seem unimportant. My thoughts were mainly on our baby growing inside and what he'd be like once he's born." Lydia thought her purchase of the water indicated her approaching labor and that the coins pouring out of the change machine symbolized delivery.

Then she added, "But the overall feeling of the dream was that I won and I didn't have to invest much at all to do it!" Later, Lydia reported giving birth to a healthy, eight-pound, two-ounce baby boy after a brief five-hour labor.

Rona, a 29-year-old choral director, also experienced happy dreams near the end of her pregnancy. Two weeks before her delivery, she submitted the following:

> It was a sunny, summer day. My husband Oliver and I were lying on a hillside watching the clouds overhead. We

were imagining seeing shapes in the clouds, the way we used to do as children. I was resting my head on Ollie's arm, feeling safe and happy. He pointed to one cloud and said, "Look at that one. It looks like a little angel or cherub." I laughed and said, "Maybe it's our baby. Wouldn't it be nice if we could just reach up and get it, and not even have to go through labor!" Ollie said, "Oh, I don't know. If it was that easy, I don't think we'd appreciate it as much." Then the cloud changed into a round ball—like a white sphere—and started coming straight down at us. I felt a little scared and said, "What's happening? Is it a UFO, or what?" and Ollie told me to hush and be still. Then the white sphere landed on my stomach and sort of spread all over my maternity skirt. Ollie was holding me tight and whispering to me not to move. Then a kind of vapor began coming out of my clothes, like white steam. My skin felt very warm but it didn't burn. Ollie told me to breathe deep and slow, Lamaze-style. I did and could feel my pelvis opening up. I had to spread my legs open and I pulled down my panties. Ollie undid my skirt and pulled it up. I felt this strong urge to bear down and push. A huge gush of water like a fountain spurted out of me. Then, there coming out between my legs was the baby. It looked just like a cherub, even had little white feathery wings. (Then I woke up. I was so happy and excited I had to wake up Ollie to tell him about it. He thought maybe my labor had started and was very relieved it was a dream.)

Rona told us that her dream of giving birth to an angelic baby descending from the clouds seemed to be a mystical, spiritual vision. "Feelings of reverence, like being in church, stayed with me for hours," she said. "Even now, just remembering it, I get goose bumps." Rona reported that her actual labor was "not as heavenly as my dreams—but not anywhere near as awful as my nightmares, either!" With Oliver's coaching, she delivered their seven-pound, nine-ounce baby girl—whom they aptly named Angela—after a "very hard, pretty fast" labor of ten hours.

Here are excerpts from a few other sweet dreams of late pregnancy:

Zena, 31-year-old secretary in her eighth month: Helping with the church Easter egg hunt . . . a tiny little boy sitting in the bushes, crying because he hadn't found any. I rocked him and calmed him. We found a huge basket bigger than he was, with all kinds of goodies, even a baby chick. . . . He squeezed the chick and it turned into a naked baby boy. We laughed and laughed!

Babs, 25-year-old librarian in her seventh month: At the lake, floating on my stomach . . . felt so light, buoyant . . . saw colorful tropical fish below . . . so happy I didn't want to wake up.

Millicent, 30-year-old homemaker, mother of a 2 year old, in her ninth month: In Rome (haven't really been there) . . . playing in the Fountain of Trevi with my son, trying to catch goldfish . . . a policeman in white uniform came and helped me deliver my baby in the water. It was a girl. He kept saying happy Italian words I couldn't understand, but I knew he was congratulating us. . . . My son held the baby. We were so happy. People were cheering and singing.

All these dreams have symbols of pregnancy and the fetus: Zena's eggs, the tiny little boy, and the baby chick; Babs's colorful tropical fish; and Millicent's goldfish in the fountain. Note also the labor and birth themes: Zena's chick turning into a baby, Babs's buoyant lake, and Millicent's actual delivery with the help of the white-uniformed policeman (an authority figure who might have symbolized her doctor or her husband). However, the overall feelings and emotional tones of these dreams remain happy and pleasurable.

Other Pleasant Dreams

You don't have to wait until the end of your pregnancy to experience sweet dreams. Everyone probably has had them, yet we are more apt to remember the nightmares; waking in fear or terror recalls stronger emotions than a relaxed, pleasant awakening.

However, sometimes nice dreams possess unusual—and truly memorable—characteristics. This is typically the case when you dream that you're flying, when you and your mate have what appear to be the same or similar visions on the same night, or when you dream of communicating with your unborn child.

FLYING DREAMS

Although a number of popular books describe the wonderful sensations of dreamers being able to fly, these nocturnal episodes are comparatively unusual. In *Creative Dreaming,* Dr. Patricia Garfield personally recalls having had as many as five or six such dreams per month. She also points out that flying dreams often precede spontaneous, lucid dreams.

Although I've taught seven pregnant women to incubate flying dreams, only three reported experiencing them spontaneously. Betsy, a homemaker with two children, had numerous dreams of flying with her entire family. Near the end of her third pregnancy, she shared the following:

> I was having a picnic at the lake with my two kids, Tiffany and Jamie, and my husband Dennis. Suddenly, the sky got dark and raindrops fell. Big waves were rising up on the lake. Dennis started packing our lunch and blanket away and I said, "Let's just take all of it and go up above the rain clouds." Tiffany and Jamie started jumping up and down and yelling, "Yeah! Let's fly, let's fly!" Dennis said we were being silly, that we couldn't really fly. I argued with him that I knew we could if we tried and he said, "You must think you're Superwoman!" Then I just grabbed his arm and took a deep breath. When I blew my breath out, we rose up about three feet off the ground. Dennis' mouth fell open. Then I reached down with the other hand and got Tiffany's hand. She held onto her brother and soon we were all up in the air. The kids were giggling. Now the rain was coming down harder. I said, "Hurry up, all of you.

Just flap your arms and we can go higher." The kids went straight up. Dennis was resisting, shaking his head and saying this was crazy. So I pulled him with me and we went up, too. I was pregnant in this dream and it was hard to pull Dennis, so I let go of him and he began to float back toward the ground. I shouted, "Flap your arms, flap your arms!" but he didn't. Then the dark cloud came between us and I couldn't see him any more. The kids and I flew around up there awhile, playing tag. It felt terrific to be so light and airy, not to feel the heavy pull of gravity now that I'm so big! Then the dark cloud disappeared so we flew back down. Dennis was sitting on our blanket with the picnic spread out. He said, "Where have you been? I'm getting hungry" and I woke up. (I felt annoyed with Dennis because he just wouldn't believe we could really fly and this resentment stayed with me quite awhile after I woke up. I used to tell him about my flying dreams, but I stopped because he would laugh at me and teased me, saying I must think I'm Mary Poppins or Tinkerbell.)

With long, curly blonde hair and a petite frame despite her large belly, Betsy possessed a somewhat elfin look. Her children were indeed lucky because she had a marvelous imagination and could easily relate to their belief in fairy tales and magic. Perhaps Dennis brought to the marriage enough skepticism and left-brain traits to help maintain a healthy balance.

Even though her husband scoffed at her flying dreams, Betsy enjoyed them tremendously. Anyone who has reported such dreams appears to derive special joy from them and generally awakens feeling happy. Although Betsy's dream indicated a few conflicts—such as her complaint that Dennis didn't share her self-confidence and the possibility that their harmonious family life (symbolized by the picnic) might be disrupted by Betsy's approaching labor and delivery (the storm and waves)—its overall tone was pleasant and carefree, typical of most flying dreams.

If you have not yet enjoyed any of these rare or unusual

consciousness experiences, you may want to attempt to incubate a flying dream. Simply follow the instructions in Chapter 7, relax deeply, and repeat to yourself as you fall asleep, "Tonight I will fly in my dreams, tonight I will fly in my dreams." Some students say they did this for two or three nights before the dream appeared, so don't be discouraged if your first attempt fails. Try again for at least two more nights.

TELEPATHIC DREAMS

Dr. Montague Ullman and Dr. Stanley Krippner, directors of one of the first sleep laboratories at the Maimonides Medical Center in New York, conducted carefully controlled experiments to test the idea that people with reportedly rare telepathic abilities could dream about a specific topic being "psychically broadcast" to them by someone else in another room.

Although the researchers did not obtain highly significant results, they found a remarkable number of individuals who consistently dreamed about symbols apparently related to the topic being "sent" to them during their sleep.

Tamari, a 33-year-old masseuse in her second pregnancy, similarly claimed to receive dream matter from her husband Bahkta. While she slept, he would sit in another room and concentrate on a photograph or illustration chosen at random from magazines Tamari had not seen. After Bahkta selected a color photograph of Vermeer's oil painting featuring a woman standing by a window with one hand on a water pitcher, Tamari reported this dream:

> I am in our kitchen, preparing soup for dinner. At the same time, I have an eye on our four-year-old daughter, Seeta, playing outside beneath the kitchen window. Using her blocks and some twigs, she's building a round temple, like one we saw on our recent trip to India, and putting her smallest baby dolls into it. I am amused as she begins

to chant like the Hindu worshippers we saw. Then I move
over to the stove to stir the soup. I notice some queer little
animals, like small mice or maybe tiny birds in the pot and
I start picking them out with some tongs. I'm puzzled,
since we're vegetarians. Then suddenly I smell smoke and
rush back to the window. Seeta's blocks are on fire. I grab
a pitcher of water off the table and throw it down onto the
flames. The water pours and pours as if it's coming out of
a hose, in a steady spray. Seeta laughs and begins to dance
around under the shower. I see there's no danger now, so
I prop the pitcher on the window sill and go outside.
Together we play under the wonderful shower.

The water pitcher in Tamari's dream seems to echo that in
the Vermeer painting being "sent" to her by Bahkta. Her
dream also has many typical pregnancy symbols: food
preparation (nurturing the unborn); a round architectural
structure (Tamari's inner space, her uterus) with baby dolls
in it (the fetus); the soup pot (again, her uterus) containing
tiny animals (fetal symbols); and the water pitcher (another
uterine symbol) pouring forth endless fluid (labor and the
waters breaking).

Tamari and her family originally came from India and
regularly practiced Hatha Yoga and spiritual meditation. It
may be that these daily routines provided them with extraordinary abilities in controlling their dreams: Tamari,
however, was the only pregnant woman I studied who reported such telepathic powers.

SYMBIOTIC DREAMS

Another type of dream indicating some sort of telepathy did
arise during my research. I call these "symbiotic dreams"
since the dreamers were nearly always the expectant parents. In six separate cases, couples envisioned similar
themes, characters, or settings, either on the same night or
two subsequent nights. In all instances, the "symbiotic"

dreamers had never before mentioned such episodes nor were the dreams incubated. These dreams occurred spontaneously; the dreamers were as surprised as I at the similarity of their experiences.

A logical explanation is that each of these couples had the same issues on their minds the nights they shared the seemingly telepathic dreams. For example, Eric and Janet's visions of boats and water described in Chapter 4 directly related to their fear that the father-to-be could not give his wife the support she needed during labor.

Another example of this type of intimate, symbiotic dreaming happened to Kate and her second husband, Dan. During her previous marriage, Kate had her tubes tied to avoid conceiving. When she and Dan wanted to have a child, her condition could not be reversed, so they opted for *in vitro* fertilization. The first six months proved quite difficult; however, by the third trimester all Kate's check-ups indicated a healthy fetus and prospects for a normal delivery. Particularly with this medical history, Kate naturally felt dependent upon Dan for emotional support. She reported the following dream as her due date approached:

> Dan and I were on the ferry to Angel Island. Then some security guards came on deck and told all the passengers there might be a bomb on board and we were hurried into lifeboats. We disembarked on Angel Island, where we were supposed to get on another ferry to take us back to San Francisco. But Dan refused, whispering to me that the crew on the return boat looked like terrorists. So we ran off into the woods. It got dark and Dan had to carry me through the underbrush until we found a path. Then we heard people behind us and we somehow knew they were the terrorists. Dan made a torch that accidentally set fire to the forest. Now both the flames and the terrorists were chasing us. Finally we got out of the woods. Looking back, we heard the terrorists screaming and knew they were dying in the forest fire. Then, we came upon an old-

fashioned wooden cradle on our path. There was a baby in it. I picked it up and hugged it. Dan said we could take it home, since we'd "come through danger and fire to get it, so now it's ours." (I woke up feeling safe and happy.)

The same night that Kate had this dream, Dan also visioned the two of them being chased through a cave and down long dark tunnels by a shadowy monster. To help them find their way, Dan made a torch: he tore up his shirt, wrapped it around a stick, and lit it. When they stumbled out of the last tunnel into the daylight, a newborn child awaited them. Dan picked it up and gave it to Kate, telling her that she deserved this infant, having gone through so much danger to reach it.

Both these beautiful dreams appear to depict Kate's medical background, with the terrorists representing the doctors involved in the numerous surgical procedures she had undergone. Dan's torch (a phallic symbol) may have stood for his masculinity, but Kate thought it also portrayed his "lighting the way" for her to have the child she wanted so intensely.

If you and your partner want to experience dreams similar in theme or content, try incubating one on a given night. Don't be discouraged if this experiment does not produce the desired results, however, because such dreams are rare. Furthermore, the inability to share symbiotic dreams in no way reflects on your closeness or bonding. These unusual dreams are only one indication of intimacy. The majority of expectant parents claim even more important ties, such as mutual emotional support and sensitivity to each other's needs and feelings.

DREAMS OF COMMUNICATING WITH YOUR BABY

Some of the women I've studied believed that in their dreams they met and talked with their unborn babies. As is the case with many unusual consciousness experiences, a method proving these reports has not yet been devised.

Pediatricians Dr. T. Berry Brazelton and Dr. Marshall Klaus tell us that most newborn infants turn their heads toward the sound of their mothers' voices, indicating a certain prenatal familiarity with that parent. Furthermore, when the newborn is fretful, the mother's singing or music she liked while pregnant frequently will have a soothing effect.

Certainly, it won't do any harm for you and your partner to talk, sing, or play peaceful music to your unborn infant. Many expectant mothers have told me that when they do these things, a very active or kicking fetus becomes calm. Also, enjoying prenatal "conversations" with your baby may make you feel more comfortable caring for it after delivery.

Programming Happy Pregnancy Dreams

If your own dreams are still upsetting or more nightmarish in quality than they are happy, there's nothing amiss: a number of concerns in your waking life continue to require your attention. Until you resolve or simply accept these issues, your dreams will reflect the same stress or anxiety.

INCUBATING SWEET DREAMS

It is possible to experience sweet dreams at any time during your pregnancy, however, by simply repeating over and over to yourself as you fall asleep, "Tonight I'll have a happy dream." This easy technique usually results in at least a temporary respite from continuous, troubling nightmares.

On other occasions, your inner self may refuse to go along with the wish to avoid anxiety-provoking issues. This happened to Cassie, a 29-year-old attorney, who complained that she awoke several times each night with horrendous nightmares. Nearly all focused on robbers and other dangerous intruders who were continually breaking into her house and threatening her with all manner of terrible deeds. Cassie did not want to understand these nightmares. "I just want to forget all about them," she insisted.

When Cassie tried to incubate a happy dream, this was the amusing result:

> Dreamed I got out of bed to check the window. Something was sticking through where it was opened at the bottom. Up close, it looked like a huge rag doll. I started pulling it into the bedroom and there seemed to be no end to it. I tugged and pulled and pulled, and pretty soon nearly the whole room was filled with this enormous stuffed cloth doll. I got out of breath. I sat down on the edge of the bed and looked at it. It was made of patches of brightly colored cloth, sewed together like a quilt. The head was as wide as my bed and had a clown's smiling face painted on it. There was a tag around its neck that said, "My name is Happy." Then the doll began to wave his arms and came to life. He rose up so his head was against the ceiling. Just the top of his body was in the room; the rest of it was hanging out the window. That big smiling mouth opened and an awful roar came out. He said, "I'm your Happy and I'm going to strangle you!" (Then the big arms began reaching for my throat and I woke up very frightened.)

After this dream, Cassie finally agreed to look at the possibility that her nightmares deserved attention rather than avoidance. She soon realized—with the group's help—that her unexpressed emotions were threatening to "strangle" her. "When I wake up from a bad dream," she told us, "I usually feel like I'm choking. I guess that's the fear I've been trying to avoid thinking about."

After some discussion, Cassie's true feelings regarding her pregnancy surfaced. In fact, she'd seriously considered abortion until her husband convinced her to have the baby. Now in her fourth month, she realized it was too late to terminate; she must endure five more months of this invasion of her body (symbolized in her dreams by intruders breaking into her home).

Once Cassie understood that these imaginary fiends reflected her resentment of pregnancy, she stopped seeing them. Some brief counseling helped her to accept her new role as a mother-to-be, and she gave birth to a healthy seven-pound, six-ounce girl. "It was the most wonderful experience of my life," she reported, "and we both love our baby so much. Now, I'm eager to have another one, and plan to do it as soon as our daughter is out of diapers."

The lesson to be learned from Cassie's attempted incubation experience is that it's probably not possible to gain total control over your dreams. One of their natural functions appears to be the resolution of problems and conflicts. Once you confront troubling issues, then the part of consciousness that dreams becomes more flexible and will reward you with more pleasant creations.

For example, 21-year-old Justine, a homemaker in her fourth month, incubated a dream with the following result:

> Dreamed I was in the back of a big empty moving van which was parked at the back entrance of the corner supermarket. I was propped up on some big pillows. A conveyor belt came from the store right up in front of me. By pushing a button I could make the belt start or stop. Along came every kind of food you can think of. I would eat what I wanted and then send the leftovers on out. It was incredible! There were juicy barbecued chickens and ribs and hot croissants from the deli. Crispy salads of all kinds. A whole shipment of luscious fruits, all washed and ready to eat. Mouth-watering candies, cookies, cakes, bread and butter. On and on. I kept on eating and never got full or tired. It was great! The smells were so wonderful and the colors were so bright, it was awesome. Then I was trying to figure out how to make the appetizers and the main courses come before the desserts (and I woke up).

When she read her dream to our group, Justine got laughs and applause. Another woman exclaimed, "I'll bet that's every pregnant woman's fantasy!" But Justine was surprised. "I watch my diet so carefully," she told us, "and I didn't think I craved foods that much until I had this dream. Then I admitted I do get cravings, but I just don't give in to them."

During our discussion of Justine's dream, it developed that she had been depriving herself of proper nutrients in order to keep from gaining too much weight. Women with cravings for the traditional ice cream and pickles usually don't get enough protein and excessively restrict their salt intake. Since Justine was only in her fourth month, not too much damage was done. She soon began following her physician's prescribed diet and later told us she no longer had cravings—nor did she dream again about stuffing herself.

Creative daydreams and affirmations. Some women simply cannot incubate dreams, despite following all the correct procedures. If you happen to be one of these, you still may create a beautiful, enjoyable daydream. Also, see the Appendix for tips on composing affirmations for overcoming negative attitudes. Both these techniques become especially helpful during the final month and weeks of pregnancy, when the waiting may seem intolerable. The ability to create and integrate positive daydreams also remains an important skill after your delivery.

PROGRAMMING HAPPY POSTPARTUM DREAMS

Following the birth of her baby boy, 34-year-old Vera wrote me the following letter:

> Our baby was in breech position and the doctor couldn't turn him, so I had C-section. I insisted on a local anesthesia so I'd be awake when he was born. Also, I practically demanded that they let me and my husband hold him right away. They did have to take him to the ICU while I got over the effects of the sedation, and I couldn't nurse him until that was all out of my system. That took 24 hours, so the first night I didn't have my baby and I was

very upset. I had this awful nightmare that my baby was kidnapped from the hospital by a woman who looked like my mother-in-law. I followed her in a taxi but she went into a fortress and I couldn't get inside. (I woke up in a panic.)

Then, she said, she created this daydream to calm herself:

It is morning and the sun is shining through the hospital windows. A nurse brings the baby to me. After she leaves, I undress him, diapers and all, and put him on my breast. I tell him, "I'll be with you always. At least, until you're big enough to leave on your own." Then, my whole family comes in and climbs onto the bed with us. I let my daughter stroke the baby while he nurses. My husband lies next to us and cuddles us both. My mother-in-law is standing there looking left out, so I invite her over too. We all have a big, loving hug.

That daydream helped me get back to sleep. Then I dreamed of almost the exact same events. Then, the next morning, my doctor actually did let me begin breastfeeding. I am so happy!

Vera's experience indicates how you can use the techniques described in this book after your baby is born. My students who return for class reunions often comment that they employ my creative daydreaming methods when feeling especially prone to "after baby blues," the symptoms you may have heard called postpartum depression.

AFTER BABY BLUES

Interestingly, those who bonded with their newborns immediately after delivery and breast-fed successfully did not report many of these postpartum symptoms. Although an anticlimactic feeling—again, caused by rapid hormonal changes—sometimes occurs after childbirth, the nursing mothers I've studied seemed to be immune to it.

It may be that women who experience postpartum depression go through a kind of grieving period. With the new baby in an intensive care unit or a nursery, the new mother possibly is subject to a sense of loss so deep that she cannot be consoled by any amount of reassurances.

If you have decided not to breast-feed your baby, it's still important for you to give him or her the bottle yourself, especially during the first week or so. This helps your baby feel bonded to you and satisfies your own deep-seated biological need to nourish your infant. You even may stave off those dreaded after baby blues.

Should you feel the syndrome emerging—usually with extreme fatigue and a tendency to cry easily—do not repress the symptoms. Instead, talk to your partner and friends who are willing to help. Try to get outside as soon as possible for a stroll or perhaps some entertainment. Incubating a dream to find out the cause of your low mood may give you additional clues. Practice your deep relaxation techniques and imagine an ideal scene in which you are happy and alert.

In conclusion, it is my hope that this book will help you, your partner, and your baby build a harmonious and rewarding future together. By learning to relax totally and deeply, you can develop skills that may protect you and your family from many stress-related discomforts and illnesses. Finally, the twin processes of sharing your dreams and learning to control them add to a more thorough understanding of your inner self; then there is no limit to what you can accomplish in all areas of your life.

More than fifty years ago, the eminent Dr. Grantley Dick-Read made these comments about the pregnant woman:

> Her mind is of even greater importance than her physical state: for motherhood is of the mind, and the body is usually subjected to the mental processes, unless any gross abnormality exists. There is a vast territory around and about maternity which is still unexplored.

It is my belief that the expectant mother's dreams and other remarkable states of consciousness are a doorway into that "vast territory," the maternal mind. By teaching you to understand your dreams and the powers of your imagination, I have mapped the location of the doorway. Now it is my hope that you will enter it, and by doing so, discover all the joys and fulfillment that expectant parents deserve.

APPENDIX

❖

Affirmations During Pregnancy

The affirmation is a positive thought derived from the reversal of a negative one. My expectant clients have used this mechanism effectively to dispel attitudes that prevent them from overcoming the six major fears of pregnancy. For example, "I hate the way my waistline is getting thicker" was reversed into "My body grows more beautiful day by day, providing a safe, warm, nourishing home for my baby," giving the woman a greater sense of control and heightened self-esteem.

After creating these positive statements, expectant mothers next relax deeply, transcend into an alpha state, and repeat affirmations to themselves over and over. New, healthier attitudes thus become integrated into their deeper consciousness.

You may wish to choose some creative thoughts listed below to change your own attitudes. If so, find a quiet time and place with no distractions; get comfortable; take several deep, cleansing breaths; and then, as you continue to breathe slowly and evenly, either repeat the affirmation of your choice or have your partner read it to you.

For fears about your baby's health

"With each breath, I enfold my baby with love, gentleness, and warmth."

"My baby is strong and healthy."

"Each breath massages my uterus with warmth. This warmth extends to my baby."

"My baby is caressed with warmth, nourishment, and health."

"I fill my body with strong, powerful love. Each breath gives life to my baby, just as it gives life to me."

For fears of being an inadequate parent

"My baby and I are in perfect harmony now. This harmony will continue after my baby is born."

"(Partner's name) and I love our baby. This love will help us to be good parents."

"My loving touch will be the most important care I can give my baby."

"Our love is a radiant light that nourishes and protects our baby. This same love will continue to surround our baby after it is born."

"We are the perfect parents for this baby."

For fears of loss of mate

"(Name of partner) loves and respects me."

"(Name) loves me even more now that I'm pregnant."

"(Name) is having this baby too. He will help me and will take care of me and our baby."

"I am strong, healthy, and beautiful."

"My sexual needs are normal and beautiful."

For fears of difficult delivery

"When my baby is ready to be born, I will relax and trust my body."

"My partner will be there for me when I'm in labor, saying the words I need to hear to help me relax and deliver my baby normally and naturally."

For fears of loss of control

"My feelings are beautiful. I am entitled to all of them."

"My emotions are not right or wrong. They are just emotions."

"I can express my feelings in appropriate ways. I can make mistakes, ask for help, and start over. I don't have to be perfect."

"When my labor begins, I will let go of any tension. There is no need for control during labor. I will allow my body's energy to deliver my baby normally and naturally."

For fears of financial burdens

"Our first priority is our baby, who will be born strong and healthy."

"I will relax deeply and let go of all fears."

"The most important thing we can give our baby is our love."

Some expectant mothers also print their favorite affirmations on large pieces of paper or cardboard and post them in spots around the house where they're most likely to read them. For example, Colleen fastened her affirmation, "My baby is growing and making my body more beautiful day by day," above her dressing table and over her kitchen sink. "It's just there," she explained, "so even when I'm not consciously thinking about it, my mind gets the message."

You may wish to create your own affirmations after reading the ones above. Since these will be in your own words, they probably will be more beneficial to you in your efforts to dispel the negative attitudes that have been keeping you from enjoying a peaceful, anxiety-free pregnancy.

INDEX